Depression: Recognition and Treatment in General Practice

GREG WILKINSON
B.Sc., M.Phil., M.B., Ch.B., F.R.C.P. (Edin), M.R.C.Psych.

SENIOR LECTURER

General Practice Research Unit, Institute of Psychiatry, De Crespigny Park, London SE5 8AF

and

HONORARY CONSULTANT PSYCHIATRIST

The Bethlem Royal and The Maudsley Hospital, Denmark Hill, Camberwell, London SE5 8AZ

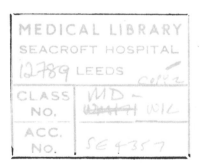
RADCLIFFE MEDICAL PRESS
OXFORD

© 1989 Radcliffe Medical Press Ltd
15 Kings Meadow, Ferry Hinksey Road, Oxford OX2 0DP

British Library Cataloguing in Publication Data

Depression: Recognition and Treatment in General Practice
1. Man. Depression. Therapy
I. Title
616.85'2706
ISBN 1 870905 16 4

Printed and bound in Great Britain
Typeset by Advance Typesetting, Oxfordshire

Contents

Foreword

DEPRESSION is a major challenge to general practice. It has an uncomfortable mortality and every year in an average group practice at least one successful suicide occurs which is potentially preventable. Last year the OPCS reported that the suicide rate rose by 22% in England and Wales. Each year one in 50 doctors will die by their own hand. Depression has a considerable morbidity. Each year a family doctor refers between two and five patients with depression to psychiatrists or other specialist agencies, and treats some 10 to 15 patients with a first attack and 30 to 70 with existing depression or relapse. Yet research shows that for every one patient diagnosed at least one other is hidden, often lurking behind an organic presentation such as headache, chest pain or backache and sometimes co-existing with organic disorders such as shingles, rheumatoid arthritis or malignancy. Depression is a fascinating intellectual challenge, ranging from a manic-depressive psychosis clearly resulting from a biochemical problem to grief, sadness and unhappiness. Providing tantalizing clues but no definitive answers to the question of why some personalities become ill from grief whilst others are enriched by the experience.

General practitioners and other primary health care workers need a good practical text that can be read in a few hours and kept in the practice or office library for easy reference. This excellent book by Dr Greg Wilkinson, a psychiatrist whose work is in general practice, in my view fills this role admirably. Although aimed at general practitioners and those in primary health care teams, it can be read to advantage by trainee psychiatrists and those consultant psychiatrists setting up in general practice for the first time. Much of the book carries practical, in-depth details emphasizing the art of treatment or 'caritas' as well as the science. Similarly, medical students spending several weeks in general practice expect a more active role nowadays and with this book and supervision they could support a patient in the initial treatment phase of depression. Patients and their relatives increasingly need to be well-informed and this text with its lucidity and absence of jargon could prove helpful in a disorder which requires compliance from the patient and support from the family. A recent trial has shown that patients with backache given an information leaflet attended less in the follow-up period than a control group with backache who were not given the leaflet. A similar concept might be tried with this book.

Dr Arthur Watts, the doyen of general practice depression studies, went away to the War from his Ibstock practice to be trained as a psychiatrist and returning to his practice wrote in 1966 'Depressive Disorders in the Community' published by John Wright which is still worth reading as a source as he covers 20 years experience of a stable Leicestershire practice of some 8000 patients. Depression is not a 20th century phenomenon. Shakespeare covered the spectrum from the melancholy *Jacques* who personifies the depressive personality ('I can suck melancholy out of a song as a weasel sucks eggs'); to the eunni of the *Merchant of Venice* ('Soothe I know not why I am so sad: It wearies me; you say it wearies you, but how I caught it, found it, or came by it, what stuff 'tis made of, whereof it is born, I am to learn.'); to Hamlet's contemplation of suicide ('or that the Everlasting had not fix'd his canon 'gainst self-slaughter! . . . To die, to sleep: To sleep per chance to dream: ay, there's the rub; . . . when he himself might his quietus make with a bare bodkin?') reveals little has changed since the Elizabethan era.

Treatment, as Dr Wilkinson has stressed, must be physical, psychological and social and the omission of any component lessens the efficacy. The very first control trial of tricyclic anti-depressants occurred in Professor Roth's Department in Newcastle in 1958 when I was an SHO completing protocols. It is ironic to look back over 30 years to see that imipramine is still a drug of choice and its successors have a lag before response; that even endogenous depression severe enough to enter the rigours of a trial in a teaching hospital had a substantial placebo response, and that it is difficult to do a double blind trial with tricyclic antidepressants until the placebo also produces a dry mouth.

Depression remains a challenge to general practice, including nurses, health visitors, psychologists, social workers and community psychiatric nurses. It is, as this book demonstrates, a field where a sensitive perceptive doctor using empathy as a diagnostic probe can sense the tear, the lack of bounce behind a familiar façade and tease out the bruised and resented inner feelings. At the same time there is room for research into prevention, better treatment, computer diagnosis, use of relatives and there are a host of other questions as yet unanswered, waiting for answers from general practice.

This book should instruct general practitioners and primary health care team workers. It is practical, direct and helpful. Few patients are more grateful than a successfully treated, previously depressed patient. This book should help doctors and patients to achieve this because as Richard Burton quoted in the Anatomy of Melancholy 'if there be a hell on earth it is to be found in a melancholy man's heart'.

DR ROBIN STEEL MBE, MB, FRCGP, DPM, Dobst,
General Practitioner, Worcester

Acknowledgements

THE rationale and structure of this book arose from the experience of preparing a guide to depression for patients and their lay helpers (Wilkinson (1989) *Depression* London: BMA).

My thanks go to Kate Martin and Gillian Nineham of Radcliffe Medical Press Ltd.

The publishers would also like to express appreciation for the financial support provided by Boots Company PLC.

1 Introduction

THIS book was conceived as a practical guide for general practitioners (GPs). It deals with the recognition of depression in patients as they present in general practice and it provides indications for appropriate, comprehensive treatment based on established and well-researched principles. The rationale for the book is that depressive illness is common in general practice, and it is both under-diagnosed and under-treated.

Although depressive illness is very common, its extent varies in different places and in different groups (Table 1.1). Surveys show that 20 – 30% of the population may suffer symptoms of depression in the course of 1 year. Most cases are mild but about 1 person in 20 will have a moderate or severe episode. Severe depression affects about 3 – 4% of the population, but only one-fifth of this group will seek medical treatment. About 1 in 50 depressives need hospital treatment.

Table 1.1: *Main sociodemographic findings*

- Women are about twice as likely as men to suffer from mild depression, but for severe depression and recurrent depression equal proportions of men and women suffer.
- Among women, the incidence and prevalence of depression vary with age—the highest rates occur in the 35 – 45 years age-group.
- The rates of depression increase with age in men.
- The incidence of depression seems highest in people belonging to socio-economic groups I and V.
- The incidence of depression is lower in married people than in single people.
- A small subset of depressives suffer from 'seasonal affective disorder' with recurrent episodes of depression in the winter months; an even smaller subset suffer from recurrent summer depressions.

The majority of depressed patients are dealt with by GPs, and depression presenting with or without anxiety constitutes the bulk of psychiatric morbidity seen in general practice.

In any one practice over a 20-year period, three quarters of the women and half the men will be seen at least once for a problem regarded by their GP as largely or wholly psychiatric in nature. In any given year, women are more likely to become depressed than men, and are less likely to recover.

The most important problem is that many patients with depression remain undiagnosed, and one of the aims of this book is to help to increase the rate of accurate diagnosis of depression by GPs. Every year a GP will treat about 30 patients for depression but may fail to recognize or be consulted by 10 times as many patients who have concealed depression.

In addition, over the course of 1 year in a notional practice of 2500 patients, 4 or 5 depressed patients will have to be seen by a psychiatrist at an outpatient clinic, 1 depressed patient will be admitted to a psychiatric hospital, 2 or 3 patients will deliberately harm themselves, and there will be 1 successful suicide attempt every 3 or 4 years.

GPs tend to view patients with depression from a different perspective to that of a psychiatrist because they usually see patients in the early stages of illness, before the full clinical picture has emerged, and in most of their patients depression is a relatively transient disorder. Moreover, the relationships of GPs with their patients are continuous, and often involve the patients' families. Thus, GPs are able to relate other aspects of patients' lives to their condition more easily than a psychiatrist. This dimension provides important advantages for the GP where treatment is concerned.

It is certainly within the scope of any GP to treat nearly all the depressive disorders, except for the most severe, and this fact has not been emphasized sufficiently in the past.

The main areas in which family doctors' management of depression can be improved are prescription of adequate doses of antidepressant, patient treatment compliance, patient supervision and recognition of depression in patients with organic disease. In between 25 and 50% of patients, there will be scope to increase the dose of antidepressant. About half the patients on antidepressants do not take the medication as prescribed and most of them will have stopped taking it altogether within a few weeks, sometimes because of side-effects but often because they do not understand the mode of action of the drug or length of treatment required.

Depressed patients on drug treatment need support, particularly when treatment begins. It is insufficient to prescribe medication and make no further arrangements. As treatment takes effect (over the course of 2 – 3 weeks), the patient may experience abrupt mood swings and there is a danger that the patient may commit suicide. It may be necessary to see the patient weekly to begin with, then, when progress is satisfactory, fortnightly, and, finally, monthly for 3 – 6 months. The exact timing of intervals depends largely on the patient's social circumstances and resources. However, it is usually advisable to inform the patient and any relatives that they can and should contact you at any time if they are worried. It is also advisable to continue to see the patient monthly for 2 – 3 months once they have recovered to check for signs of relapse. It is possible to give a focus to these appointments by asking the patient to keep a diary describing their moods and activities since the last appointment.

Specialist help may be required for patients in whom the diagnosis is in doubt, there is a high risk of suicide being attempted or progress is slow despite appropriate treatment. The majority of disturbed patients, in particular, those who have psychological or motor retardation, agitation or psychotic symptoms, such as hallucinations and delusions, will need to be referred to a psychiatrist. In disturbed patients, the illness is obvious to all concerned, including relatives, who are often pleased to have specialist advice and treatment. Patients with depression who live alone, or take excess alcohol, are also particulary vulnerable and usually require extra social support as part of their treatment.

2 Recognizing Depressive Illness

DEPRESSIVE illness is a persistent exaggeration of the everyday feelings that accompany sadness. It is a disturbance of mood, of variable severity and duration, that is frequently recurrent, and accompanied by a variety of physical and mental symptoms, involving thinking, drive and judgement.

Depressive illness is usually recognized by the affected individual or close family and friends when the symptoms become severe or last for too long. In practice, incipient or established depressive illness is recognized by eliciting several of the following symptoms:

- *persistent*, low, miserable mood;
- sleep disturbance;
- lack of enjoyment or pleasure in usual activities;
- reduced energy and weariness;
- loss of appetite or weight (rarely gain);
- impaired efficiency;
- self-reproach and guilt;
- inability to concentrate and make decisions;
- distinctive posture and gesture.

Anxiety, irritability, agitation and retardation are often present.

In severe depression, the above characteristics are present with greater intensity and may be accompanied by:

- suicidal ideas, plans or acts;
- failure to eat or drink;
- delusions and/or hallucinations.

In a primary care setting, prevention of morbidity should be the main goal, and for this reason it is inappropriate to think that a threshold of five or six of the above symptoms should be present before a diagnosis of depression can be made.

The goal should be to recognize and treat incipient depressions. The longer a patient's depression persists, especially when it is experienced daily, the more likely it is that depressive illness is present. Most episodes of depression lasting for more than 2 weeks become depressive illnesses.

Diagnosis of depression

A diagnosis is made based on the type, duration, persistence and number of characteristic symptoms present. A patient's depressed mood is particularly likely to be pathological if its pervasiveness, duration and severity exceed what might otherwise be regarded as normal in the circumstances or its causes appear insufficient to explain the degree of disorder.

In its more severe forms, the sadness and misery experienced in depressive illness is disabling and out of proportion to any stress that a person has previously endured.

The typical acute presentations of depression are given in Table 2.1, and the typical clinical presentations of established depression are illustrated in Case Histories I and II. The symptoms of depression are listed in Table 2.2.

Table 2.1: *Typical acute presentations of depression.*

- Normal activity disrupted: unable to cope with daily duties; unable to go to work; unable to get out of bed.
- Vague physical symptoms: tiredness; loss of appetite and weight; insomnia.
- Difficulty coping: alcohol abuse; drug abuse; violent impulses or behaviour.
- Worried family and friends: frustration; loss of sympathy; guilt.
- Suicide: thoughts; plans; attempts.

Case History: I

Jim found that he was beginning to feel isolated and lonely, even when his friends and family were around. He could no longer feel affection for his loved ones and he rejected their attempts to comfort him. Increasingly, he found it difficult to cry; in any case, tears no longer brought relief. Gradually, his energy waned and he lost interest in things; talking and concentration became an effort. He found himself thinking a great deal about the past, and unpleasant memories returned to upset him. He started to feel restless, agitated and irritable and sometimes he became very anxious. He was always gloomy: pessimism and hopelessness were ever present.

Table 2.2: *Symptoms of depression.*

Mood	Thinking	Drive	Physical	Judgement
Sadness	Loss of interest	Wish to escape	Feeling run down	Delusions:
Misery	Lack of self-esteem	Withdrawal	Tired	typically of guilt,
Gloom	Sensitivity	Feeling of being	Aches	worthlessness or nihilism
Despondency	Sense of inadequacy	in a rut	Pains	and of hypochondriasis,
Anxiety and tension	Sense of apathy	Activities seem dull	Loss of appetite	e.g. that brain or bowels
Lack of enjoyment	Sense of futility	or meaningless	Loss of weight	have rotted
Lack of satisfaction	Inability to cope	Desire to seek refuge	Sleep disturbance	
Loss of affection	Difficulty making		Loss of sexual appetite	Hallucinations:
Weeping	decisions		Fatigue	typically auditory,
Labile mood	Shame		Inability to relax	of someone talking
Temper	Hopelessness		Autonomic symptoms	to the patient, the
Irritability	Self-blame		Agitation	content being negative,
	Worthlessness		Motor retardation	e.g. "you are dying
	Forgetfulness and		Constipation	of cancer/AIDS"
	inability to			
	concentrate			

Adapted from Wilkinson (1989) *Depression* London: BMA.

Case History: II

Barbara was miserable, particularly in the mornings. Her sleep pattern had changed: she was finding it difficult to get off to sleep in the evening and she was waking up in the early hours, unable to get back to sleep. She worried increasingly about her health. Her mother had died of breast cancer and she began to think that she would die from the same cause. She was off her food and had lost half a stone in weight in the past month. She had taken time off work because she was unable to cope and she began thinking that she was worthless. Feelings of guilt occupied her thoughts. She could no longer bear her husband's embrace. Barbara criticized her performance as a wife and mother and blamed herself for bringing shame upon her family. Life no longer seemed worth living.

Distinction between anxiety and depression

Studies based on psychiatric hospital patients show that anxiety and depression are separate and distinct, and that there is little overlap between the two. The reverse is true with studies conducted in general practice and in the community, where there is a high correlation between measures of anxiety and depression. This does not mean that 'pure' anxiety and 'pure' depression do not exist, but that many patients experience both symptoms. Although psychiatrists distinguish between the concepts of anxiety and depression, patients do not appear to do so.

Somatization

Although depression, anxiety, worry and fatigue are the commonest symptoms of depressive disorders in general practice, half of all such patients complain of somatic symptoms, precipitated, exacerbated or maintained by psychological factors, and sleep disturbance. Among the commonest somatic symptoms reported are: headache, backache, other regional pains, and dizzy spells. Other somatic symptoms include asthenia, palpitations, dyspnoea, nausea and sweating. Around one-quarter of these patients are excessively concerned with various other aspects of their bodily function.

Missed depression

Much depressive disorder is missed in primary care. It is claimed that GPs do not recognize between 30 and 50% of patients with psychiatric morbidity presenting to them.

Table 2.3: *Factors responsible for failure to detect depression.*

- Depressions masked by presentation in terms of *somatic symptoms.*
- Depressions judged to be *demoralization reaction* to medical problem.
- Depressions *missed* through incomplete diagnostic work-up.
- Depressions *minimized* relative to physical disease.
- Depressions *misdiagnosed* as a *dementia* in the elderly.
- Depressions *misperceived* as a *negative attitude.*

Adapted from Derogatis & Wise (1989) *Anxiety and Depressive Disorders in the Medical Patient* Washington, DC: American Psychiatric Press, Inc.

Some of the practical problems surrounding the diagnosis and classification of depressive disorders were poignantly illustrated by Dr Arthur Watts in a revealing look back at his experience of psychiatry in general practice in the 1940s (*Bulletin of the Royal College of Psychiatrists, 1986*):

'In those days I had a complete blind spot as regards depression. I had heard about melancholia, and Hector McPhail had showed us cases of a woman who could not stop weeping and an old man verging on a stupor. When a man came to see me complaining of constipation I gave him a good physical examination; I even referred him for a bowel X-ray which was negative. Once I had the hospital report I saw my patient, and gave him a clean bill of health and told him he had nothing to worry about. He went straight home and put his head in a gas oven. Even when I heard the news, it never dawned on me that I had missed a classic case of depression; indeed I felt rather indignant that he hadn't believed me.'

Understanding psychiatric morbidity

Conspicuous psychiatric morbidity is a term used to refer to that proportion of total psychiatric morbidity recognized by doctors. The difference between total and conspicuous psychiatric morbidity is an index of the level of detection of psychiatric disorder.

Factors affecting detection are the GP's personality, training, attitudes and interview techniques. Additional factors are the pattern of the patient's presenting symptoms and sociodemographic characteristics. Women, the middle-aged and those who are separated or divorced are more likely to be identified as having conspicuous morbidity.

Hidden psychiatric morbidity is a term used to refer to that proportion of psychiatric morbidity not recognized by doctors. Patients with hidden morbidity have as many symptoms as those with conspicuous illness, and they do not have a better prognosis.

Patients who are unlikely to have their depressive illness detected typically present to their GP with physical symptoms and do not volunteer their psychological symptoms unless the GP makes a direct enquiry. If the GP is made aware of depressive illnesses, patients are more likely to get better quickly and to have fewer symptoms a year later at follow-up.

For every 2 patients with psychiatric disorder recognized by a GP, a third patient with a psychiatric disorder will be missed. GPs vary widely in their ability to identify psychiatric illness correctly and consequently in the amount of hidden morbidity they miss.

Diagnostic bias and accuracy

Bias is the tendency to make or avoid making psychiatric diagnoses. GPs with a high bias have a low threshold for making these diagnoses, and vice versa. It has been found that there is no correlation between a GP's estimate of conspicuous psychiatric morbidity and the probable presence of morbidity by screening, therefore it can be concluded that conspicuous psychiatric morbidity is a measure of bias. GPs with a high bias tend to ask many psychiatric questions and questions about the patient's home life. They are empathic and sensitive to verbal questions relating to psychological distress. However, they are no more accurate in their assessments than GPs who have a low bias.

Accuracy is the overall ability to make diagnoses of psychiatric disturbances which are in keeping with the patient's symptoms. It is possible to account for a large proportion of the variation in accuracy among GPs in terms of personalities, academic ability and interview technique (Table 2.4). GPs who are more accurate are likely to have high scores on scales measuring positive self-regard and responsiveness to personal needs and feelings. They are also more likely to possess higher qualifications and have greater knowledge of clinical medicine. GPs using directive interview techniques are also likely to be more accurate, possibly because they have a better idea of the likely goal of their questioning.

GPs who make many psychiatric diagnoses are no more accurate than those who make few such diagnoses.

Table 2.4: *Interviewing behaviour related to accuracy of diagnosis of depression.*

Early in interview

- Establish good eye contact.
- Clarify the patient's presenting complaint.
- Use direct questions for physical complaints.
- Use open-to-closed questioning style.

During interview

- Use an empathic style.
- Be sensitive to verbal and non-verbal cues.
- Avoid reading notes in front of the patient.
- Cope well with over-talkativeness.
- Do not concentrate on the patient's past history.

Adapted from Goldberg and Huxley (1980) *Pathways to Psychiatric Care*. Tavistock Publications, London.

Table 2.5: *Cues for the recognition of depression.*

- Patient volunteers: 'I am depressed'.
- Symptom(s) associated with depression.
- Physical symptoms without physical cause.
- Recurrent presentation of children by patient.
- Doctor feels depressed by patient.
- Doctor thinks patient is depressed.
- Fat case-record.
- Patients unduly troubled by symptoms.
- Patients consulting without a change in clinical status.
- Patients seemingly dissatisfied with their care.

Natural history of depression

1 Those who experience their symptoms in response to an identifiable life event, and whose depression remits rapidly and often spontaneously. This may account for up to 50% of the depressed individuals in the community.

2 Depressed individuals whose depression lasts longer and recurs more frequently.

3 Chronically depressed individuals who might be regarded as having a depressive personality.

Course of depressive illnesses

Depression can affect people of all ages, but severe depression usually begins at around the age of 30 – 40 years.

In the beginning, when the onset of depressive illness is fairly sudden, symptoms can develop in 1 – 2 weeks, although it is more usual for the rate to be 2 or 3 times slower. The commonest symptoms are depressed mood, anxiety and loss of interest; sleep difficulties, loss of appetite, lack of energy, fatigue and suicidal thoughts soon follow.

After 3 – 5 months, patients tend to seek medical help because they can no longer cope. By this time, the illness is often severe, and profoundly depressed mood, guilty thoughts and suicidal ideas are clearly present. In the most severe depressive illnesses, hallucinations and delusions develop.

If depressive illness has become established, it tends to last for months, perhaps even years, without treatment.

Remission nearly always occurs, particularly in younger patients. About one-third of patients have only one attack of depression in their lives, with return to normal premorbid functioning. About 50% of patients who have a single episode of severe depression will eventually have a second episode, which occurs 2 – 5 years after the first. The episodes tend to become more frequent and to last for longer in older people.

In the most severe cases, relapse is likely after recovery in about three-quarters of affected individuals. Chronic, persistent or fluctuating symptoms, social difficulties and impairments occur in up to one-third of patients.

The course of recurrent depressions is highly variable: some patients have episodes separated by many years of normal functioning, some are subject to clusters of episodes, and others experience increasingly frequent episodes as they grow older. Overall functioning usually returns to the premorbid level between episodes. In one-fifth to one-third of cases, there is a chronic course with considerable residual symptoms and social impairment. About 15% of severely depressed people eventually commit suicide.

The GP's perspective

The GP has a different perspective of depressive illness to that promoted by the classifications provided by psychiatrists (see Appendix to this chapter, p.16). GPs have a continuous relationship with their patients and, often, the patients' families. Also, the features of depressive morbidity in general practice are not well-defined, because there is a high incidence of transient disorders and illness often seen in its early stages before the full clinical picture has developed. Furthermore, the morbidity seen in primary care is often a combination of psychological, physical and social elements.

Table 2.6: *International classification of health problems in primary care-2-defined diagnostic criteria.*

Depressive disorder (neurotic depression)

Inclusion in this rubric requires satisfaction of the following critera.

1   Absence of psychosis.

2   Presence of three of the following symptoms

   i   sadness or melancholy out of proportion to psychosocial stress;
   ii   suicidal thoughts or attempt;
   iii   indecisiveness, decrease in interest in usual activities or slow thinking;
   iv   feelings of worthlessness, self-reproach or inappropriate or excessive guilt;
   v   early morning waking, hypersomnia and morning tiredness;
   vi   anxiety, irritability and agitation.

Table 2.6 *continued.*

Affective psychoses

Inclusion in this rubric requires satisfaction of all of the following criteria.

1 Disorder predominantly in the area of mood, showing either severe depression or marked elation and expansiveness, or alternation of the two, distinguishable from the usual range of emotion.

2 Disorder of such a degree that it grossly impedes the ability of the patient to meet the ordinary demands of life.

3 If psychosis is unipolar, disorder of thought (delusions, hallucinations or paranoid state).

It is necessary to appreciate that the majority of patients suffering from psychiatric morbidity presenting in general practice or identified in community surveys fall within a single broad category—depression with or without associated anxiety. However, it is well known that there is wide disagreement among GPs with respect to the diagnosis of depression. Differences are most apparent at the minor end of the spectrum of depressive morbidity, particularly where the distinction between illness, distress and 'disgust with life in general' remains unresolved.

Recognition of depression in adults

Patients in whom psychiatric disorder is missed often present with physical disorder, either because a new and serious physical symptom has appeared leading to depression which the GP overlooks or because a chronic physical symptom is persisting and the underlying depression is missed.

Depressed patients tend to present with physical symptoms for three main reasons.

1 There is the common belief that doctors deal with physical disorders and only physical symptoms should be presented.

2 Physical and psychiatric disorders frequently co-exist. Thus, the exacerbation of a chronic physical disorder may be a useful warning that there is a concurrent psychiatric disorder.

3 There is a stigma associated with psychiatric disorder and the patient may wish to deal with the GP in physical terms.

Many patients do not recognize (or cannot convey) the nature of their depression. In one general practice study, less than half the depressives regarded themselves as depressed and only a very small percentage had consulted the GP primarily for depression.

Patients with unrecognized depression may be more difficult to identify because they are less likely to admit to it or complain of it and they appear and behave in a less depressed way, although they are likely to have had their symptoms for longer than those patients whose depression is more easily recognized and to be as handicapped.

Recognition of depression in the elderly

GPs have little difficulty in recognizing depression in the elderly, but recognition does not necessarily lead to treatment with antidepressants or specialist referral. This may be because of the expectations that depression is part and parcel of old age.

At first, an elderly depressed person may appear to be difficult, complaining, querulous, irritable and demanding, and may not mention any depression. He or she may appear confused, forgetful, withdrawn and out of touch, seemingly demented, when really the problem is depression.

Table 2.7: *Discrimination of depression from dementia in the elderly.*

Clinical features	Depression	Dementia
Onset	Relatively rapid	Insidious
Cognitive impairment	Fluctuating	Constant
Memory/comprehension	Will respond to treatment	Progressive/no response to treatment
Sense of distress	Yes	No/blunting
Self-image	Negative	Unaffected
Somatic symptoms	Typical	Atypical except sleep

Adapted from Derogatis & Wise (1989) *Anxiety and Depressive Disorders in the Medical Patient* Washington, DC: American Psychiatric Press, Inc.

Recognition of depression in adolescence

Inner turmoil, misery and low self-esteem occur frequently in adolescence. GPs may be reluctant to diagnose depression because of the view that depressive feelings are so common in teenagers. In fact, psychiatric disturbance occurs about as often in this age-group as in any other age-group.

Recognition of depression in children

Prepubertal depression occurs and may herald depression in later life.

Depression is common in both the short and the long term in children who have been sexually abused. Thus, depression may be an important behavioural warning of child abuse for the GP.

It is important to consider the possibility of depression in a young child and distinguish this from sadness in response to difficulties.

The characteristic features of depression in children are anxiety, sleep disturbance, irritability, suicidal thoughts, eating disturbance, school refusal, phobias, abdominal complaints, obsessions and hypochondriasis.

Conclusion

Much of the variation in the reported prevalence of depressive disorders in general practice is due to differences in classification and diagnosis. GPs could achieve much by simply heightening their awareness of depression and its somatic presentations. Early recognition and the institution of adequate treatment should lead to great improvements in the quality of life of many patients who might otherwise suffer needlessly.

Appendix: *Diagnostic criteria for depression* (adapted from the *American Psychiatric Association's Diagnostic and Statistical Manual (DSM-III-R)*)

Major depressive episode

At least 5 of the symptoms listed below should present during the same 2 week period, most of them occurring nearly every day, representing a change from previous functioning. At least 1 of the symptoms should be either depressed mood or loss of interest or pleasure. Symptoms clearly due to physical conditions, mood-incongruent delusions or hallucinations and incoherence are not included.

Symptoms

1 Depressed mood.

2 Markedly diminished interest or pleasure in all, or almost all, activities.

3 Significant weight loss or weight gain when not dieting (e.g. more than 5% of bodyweight in 1 month), or a decrease or increase in appetite.

4 Insomnia or hypersomnia.

5 Psychomotor agitation or retardation.

6 Fatigue or loss of energy.

7 Feelings of worthlessness or excessive or inappropriate guilt (may be delusional, not merely self-reproach or guilt about being sick).

8 Diminished ability to think or concentrate, or indecisiveness.

9 Recurrent thoughts of death (not just fear of dying), recurrent suicidal ideation without a specific plan or a suicide attempt or a specific plan for committing suicide.

It is not possible to establish that an organic factor initiated and maintained the disturbance, which is not a normal reaction to the death of a loved one. At no time during the disturbance have there been delusions or hallucinations for as long as 2 weeks in the absence of prominent mood symptoms, and the condition is not superimposed on schizophrenia or similar psychotic disorder.

Seasonal pattern

There is a regular temporal relationship between the onset of an episode of bipolar disorder or recurrent major depression in a particular 60-day period (for example, regular episodes of depression between the beginning of October and the end of November). Cases in which there is an obvious effect of seasonally related psychosocial factors are not included.

Full remissions (or a change from depression to mania or hypomania) also occurs within within a particular 60-day period (for example, depression is absent from mid-February to mid-April).

There have been at least 3 episodes of mood disturbance in 3 separate years that demonstrated this temporal seasonal relationship, and at least 2 of the years were consecutive.

Seasonal episodes of mood disturbance outnumber any non-seasonal episodes of such disturbance by more than 3:1.

Bipolar disorder

Current or most recent episode involves the full symptomatic picture of both manic and major depressive episodes except for the duration requirement of 2 weeks for depressive symptoms, intermixed or rapidly alternating every few days. Prominent depressive symptoms lasting at least 1 full day.

Dysthymia (depressive neurosis)

Depressed mood for most of the day, more days than not, for at least 2 years. While depressed at least 2 of the following must be present:

1 poor appetite or overeating;

2 insomnia or hypersomnia;

3 low energy or fatigue;

4   low self-esteem;

5   poor concentration or difficulty making decisions;

6   feelings of hopelessness.

During a 2-year period of the disturbance, the patient is never without symptoms for more than 2 months at a time.

No evidence of a major depressive episode during the first 2 years of the disturbance. The patient has never had a manic episode and the disorder is not superimposed on a chronic psychotic disorder, nor can it be established that an organic factor initiated and maintained the disturbance.

3 Types of Depression

DEPRESSIVE illnesses vary in severity. Milder forms of depression are often called 'neurotic' or 'reactive' depression, whereas the more severe forms of the illness are called 'manic-depressive psychosis' or 'endogenous' depression. Milder illnesses are much more common in general practice.

There are also a variety of terms to describe different types of depression, although these do not necessarily further our understanding of the condition. Many, if not most, of these terms are more useful for the purposes of research and administration rather than clinical practice.

Classification based on cause

Reactive and endogenous depression

In reactive depression, symptoms are thought to be responses to external stress, whereas in endogenous depression symptoms seem to occur independently of environmental causes. In many cases, this distinction does not seem to be clear. Precipitating events have been shown to precede both types of illness and the existence of two distinct symptom clusters has not been confirmed.

Endogenous depression is defined in terms of sadness, social withdrawal, loss of libido, anorexia/weight loss, retardation/agitation, early morning wakening, guilt, loss of pleasure, diurnal variations of mood, and mood unresponsive to the environment. This mood is qualitatively distinct from normal sadness.

Primary and secondary depression

The aim in this classification is to separate secondary depressions, i.e. those due to other psychiatric or physical illnesses and drug and alcohol abuse, from primary depressions (those that do not have such causes). This classification is mainly used for research purposes.

Classification based on symptoms

Neurotic and psychotic depression

The distinction between these conditions is not very obvious, with many patients having features of both types. Nevertheless, this is probably the classification in widest clinical use.

Neurotic depression is characterized by disproportionate depression which has usually followed a distressing experience. There is often preoccupation with the emotional trauma that preceded the illness, e.g. loss of an ideal, a loved one or a treasured possession. Anxiety is also frequently present; mixed states of anxiety and depression are included in this category. Neurotic depression excludes delusions or hallucination among its features.

Manic-depressive psychoses are usually recurrent disorders in which there is a severe disturbance of mood (mostly a combination of depression and anxiety but also sometimes elation and excitement) which may be accompanied by one or more of the following: disturbed attitude to self, perplexity, delusions, and disorders of behaviour and of perception (occasionally including hallucinations). When any of the above are present, these are all in keeping with the patient's prevailing mood. There may also be a strong, often unexpressed, tendency to suicide.

The distinction between depressive neurosis and manic-depressive psychosis should be based upon the degree of depression and the presence or absence of other neurotic or psychotic characteristics, and upon the degree of disturbance of the patient's behaviour. Mild disorders of mood may be included under the category manic-depressive psychoses if the symptoms match closely the descriptions given.

Synthesis

In the past depression has been subdivided into 'reactive' depression, i.e. occurs in response to adversity, and 'endogenous' depression, which was thought to be unrelated to environmental circumstances. These terms are gradually being replaced by neurotic (instead of reactive) and psychotic (instead of endogenous). This is because depressed patients are classified according to the symptoms that they display (i.e. neurotic symptoms or psychotic symptoms), whereas the older terms refer to aetiology. The pattern of symptomatology labelled 'endogenous depression' is not uninfluenced by external circumstances as was once believed, since life events have been found to be an important precipitant.

There has long been a debate about the nature of and relationship between neurotic and psychotic depression. Are there two distinct kinds of depression, or do they represent two ends of a continuum? Can depressed patients be reliably classified into different subgroups? However there is a general agreement that there are two different types of depression, and that there is a distinct group of patients suffering from psychotic depression. Neurotic depression, however, is not generally regarded as a disease entity, but is thought to be continuously distributed in the population (like hypertension).

Clinically, two questions need to be asked, first, 'is the patient suffering from psychotic depression?' and second, 'to what extent is he suffering from neurotic depression?'

Classification by course and time of life

Unipolar and bipolar depression

Unipolar depression is used to refer to those depressions that occur alone, unassociated with manic illness. In bipolar disorders, episodes of depression and mania occur alternately or together. There is some overlap between patients in these two groups; some patients with unipolar depression are potential cases of bipolar illness which has not yet been revealed. It is doubtful that the groups differ in symptoms or in their response to treatment.

Depressive disorders in later life

There is no longer thought to be a clear distinction between depression in the elderly and that in younger people, either in relation to symptoms or treatment response.

Classification in practice

The *severity* of the depression can be described as mild, moderate or severe. The *type of episode* may be depressed, manic or mixed. *Special features* can be described, such as neurotic and psychotic symptoms, agitation and retardation. The *course* may be uni- or bipolar, and the *cause* may be reactive or endogenous, usually a combination of both is important.

Other syndromes

Bereavement reactions

Typically, the grief following bereavement consists of three main phases:

1   emotional blunting lasting from a few hours to a few weeks;

2   mourning, with intense yearning and distress, autonomic features, a sense of futility, anorexia, restlessness or irritability, preoccupation with the deceased (including transient hallucinatory experiences), guilt and even denial of the fact of death;

3   acceptance and re-adjustment take place several weeks after the onset of mourning.

Grief usually lasts for an average of 3 – 6 months, but the timing is very variable.

Atypical grief

Atypical grief may consist of:

1   chronic grief, leading to a typical depressive illness;

2   inhibited or delayed grief;

3   grief with psychiatric complications.

Atypical or masked depression

These unsatisfactory terms are occasionally used when depression is thought to underlie unexplained physical and mental disorders or otherwise inexplicable behaviour, e.g. chronic pain, hypochondriasis, psychosomatic or conversion disorders, pseudodementia, some anxiety states, and shoplifting in middle-aged women.

Postnatal depression

It is usual for women to undergo emotional disturbance, especially transient depression and weeping ('the blues'), at some time within the first 10 days after childbirth. It often lasts for 1 or 2 days and then passes. This is not the first sign of postnatal depression.

About 2 in every 1000 childbirths are complicated by the development of serious mental illness, three-quarters of which are postnatal depressive illnesses. Postnatal depressive illness may take up to 3 months or more after the baby is born to develop. It can be mild or severe, and the symptoms are identical to those of other depressive illnesses but there are the added problems of tiredness and having a baby to look after. It is usually of relatively short duration and the woman has a good prognosis. The risk of recurrence after a succeeding pregnancy is about 1 in 7.

Depressive personality

Depressive personality is characterized by a lifelong tendency to persistent gloom and despondency, usually resulting in a degree of social disability that rebounds on the individual or close family and friends. Sometimes, such individuals also experience periods of elevated mood or marked mood swings between depression and elation.

Depression and alcohol

Depressed people commonly turn to alcohol because it seems to provide temporary relief from unpleasant feelings of tension and unhappiness. However, alcohol abuse causes severe damage not only emotionally and socially but also to the family. It is also a cerebral depressant that inevitably provokes or prolongs depression.

Depression and aging

Old age is a time of increasing vulnerability to depression. Depression in the elderly may be obscured by physical illness and handicaps such as deteriorating eyesight, deafness and memory loss.

In those aged 65 years or over, the incidence of depression in men is similar to that in women. Genetic disposition becomes less important with increasing age at onset of depression. Life-events are particularly important causes of depression in the elderly. Other predisposing factors include forced early retirement, poverty and ill health. Cognitive impairment may be present, resulting in a three-way interaction between perception, mood and behaviour.

There is an age-related decrease in brain amines, and Parkinson's disease, with dopamine depletion, is associated with an increased risk of depression. Neurophysiological changes also play a part.

The prognosis can be poor; in one study, it was found that up to two-thirds of depressed elderly patients were unchanged, worse or dead 1 year after diagnosis. Factors contributing to this prognosis included psychotic illness with depressive delusions, physical illness, housing difficulties and low income.

4 Causes of Depressive Illness

THE precise cause of depression is not known. There is an important genetic element in the predisposition to depression, and unpleasant life-events and some physical illnesses play a part in precipitating and maintaining depression through biochemical and psychological mechanisms.

Genetic factors

Family, twin and adoption data are consistent and provide compelling evidence that genes make an important contribution to typical or severe forms of depression. Theories about the mode of this genetic inheritance are conflicting, and the search for 'genetic markers' has so far been unsuccessful.

Genes and environment

In manic-depressive illness, the proportion of variance contributed by genes is greater than 80%, with family environment accounting for less than 10%. In neurotic depression, the proportion of variance contributed by genes is less than 10% and that by family environment over 50%.

Family studies

Well-defined manic-depressive illness is more common in the relatives of patients than in the general population. Among first-degree relatives of patients with bipolar depressive illnesses (having episodes of mania and depression, or mania alone), there is an excess of both bipolar and unipolar depressive illness (recurrent episodes of depression only). Relatives of patients with unipolar depressive disorder have an increased risk of unipolar disorder only.

Morbid risk

The morbid risk of depressive disorder in the first-degree relatives (children, siblings and parents) of affected patients ranges from

6 to 40%. Much of the variance can be accounted for by differing diagnostic practices, but there may also be differences in the lifetime risk of depression in different populations. It has also been suggested that there may be a secular change in rates of depression with increases in lifetime prevalence evident among some younger cohorts.

Using strict diagnostic criteria, the lifetime risk for unipolar depression is about 3% and that for bipolar depression is under 1%, and both are strongly familial. The risk in first-degree relatives of bipolar depressed patients is about 20%, whereas that in unipolar patients' relatives is about 10%.

Twin and adoption studies

Monozygotic concordance rates are up to 5 times as great as dizygotic concordance rates, evidence that supports the importance of genetic factors. There is a stronger genetic contribution in bipolar disorder when compared with unipolar disorder. There is an overall concordance of 70% in monozygotic twins versus 20% in dizygotic twins when the patient has a bipolar disorder, whereas the concordance in monozygotic twins is 50% and 25% in dizygotic twins when the patient has a unipolar disorder.

Life stress

Death of a loved one, loss of a job, moving house and other major stresses have been implicated as causes of depression. The reaction is often delayed, occurring some months after the event has taken place. Adverse life-events tend to be clustered in the 6 – 12 months before the onset of depression. There appears to be an increase in the occurrence of depression after the most stressful types of life-events. Threatening types of life-events bring forward the onset of depression.

Interestingly, depression seems to be as common among the relatives of patients whose illness is not neurotic/reactive as it is among the relatives of probands whose depression is associated with threatening life-events or chronic difficulties. Also, the frequency of reported life-events is significantly increased among the relatives of depressives when compared with that of the general population. Within families, exposure to life-events shows only a weak association with depression. These findings suggest that part of the association between life-events and depression seems to be due to the fact that both show familial aggregation.

However, it should be borne in mind that patients with depression may tend to remember and report more negative life-events, and the impact of any event upon a particular person is difficult to predict.

Vulnerability factors

The following factors were found to increase the frequency of depression in working class young women in Inner London if they had also experienced a threatening life-event or major difficulties.

- Loss of mother before the age of 11 years.
- Three or more children under the age of 14 years at home.
- Lack of an intimate confiding relationship.
- Unemployment.
- Other chronic difficulties.

Vulnerability factors are thought to increase the likelihood of depression in the presence of provoking life-events, but they are not considered as causes of depression in themselves. A confiding relationship and a job could therefore be factors which protect against depression.

Low social class was found to be associated with a higher incidence of minor depressive illness in young women in Inner London. It probably acts as a vulnerability factor that lowers the threshold for depression in the face of various types of adversity.

Women are more likely to suffer from both mild and severe depression than men. The reason for this is not clear, but it is possible that circumstances associated with hormonal changes (postnatal mental illness, premenstrual syndrome), exposure to more chronic stressors and different coping styles are involved.

Coping with transition

'Psychosocial transition' occurs when an individual has to give up one set of assumptions about the world and adopt another, i.e. adopt a new way of looking at life. This might apply to bereavement, childbirth, changes of occupation, retirement and migration. It is the individual's capacity to cope with transition that determines whether or not symptoms will occur, a process of readjustment analogous to coping with bereavement.

Brain and body chemistry

There are over 40 neurotransmitters in the human central nervous system. Two of these have been the subject of special study in depression: serotonin and noradrenaline. In early studies, both were shown to be important in depressed patients, where their metabolism was noticeably decreased.

Serotonin

Hypofunction or hyperfunction of the serotonergic system may be a primary deficit in depression. In the hypofunction hypothesis, it is suggested that depression is caused by decreased availability and function of the serotonergic system. Thus, antidepressants exert a therapeutic effect by increasing synaptic serotonin availability and neurotransmission.

In the hyperfunction hypothesis, it is proposed that serotonin neurotransmission is increased in depression, presumably as a consequence of hyposensitive postsynaptic serotonin receptors.

In patients with manic-depressive/psychotic but not neurotic/reactive depression, serotonin uptake is reduced. As the depression is alleviated, platelet uptake of serotonin returns to normal. However, it is thought that many antidepressants reduce serotonin uptake and amitriptyline may work by altering the responsiveness of the serotonin receptors.

It is premature to draw any conclusions about the aetiological significance of serotonin dysfunction in depression; to do so would be to ignore complex functional interactions between the serotonin system and other neurotransmitter systems, for example the role of serotonin in the mediation of antidepressant effects on the noradrenergic system.

Noradrenaline

Uncertainty also surrounds the role of noradrenaline in depression. It plays a major role in controlling activation throughout the brain and body, and seems to be depleted in depressive illnesses.

In depressed patients, there is an increase in the number and sensitivity of the presynaptic receptors that suppress the release of noradrenaline into the synapse. These biochemical changes take time both to develop and to be corrected which is part of the reason why antidepressants do not act immediately suggesting that the delay in onset of action is inevitable.

Women

In women, the complex hormonal changes associated with menstruation, childbirth and the menopause are thought to increase the risk of depression but at present our understanding of the processes involved is limited.

Physical illness

Depression may occur as a psychological response to severe physical illnesses and chronic disabling conditions. However, some conditions also act as specific causes (see Table 4.1).

Table 4.1: *Physical causes of depression.*

● Neurological diseases:	Parkinson's disease multiple sclerosis stroke epilepsy dementia
● Malignant diseases:	lung cancer brain tumours cancer of the pancreas
● Endocrine diseases:	hypothyroidism Cushing's syndrome Addison's disease
● Kidney disease:	kidney failure kidney dialysis
● Anaemia:	iron deficiency folate deficiency vitamin B_{12} deficiency

Table 4.1: *continued.*

● Infections:	influenza and postinfluenza
	hepatitis
	glandular fever
	brucellosis
	shingles
● Side-effects of drug treatment:	methyldopa
	corticosteroids
	L-dopa
	diuretics
	barbiturates
	reserpine
● Drug withdrawal:	benzodiazepine tranquillizers
	amphetamines
	alcohol

Adapted from Wilkinson (1989) *Depression* London: BMA.

The period immediately after childbirth is also strongly associated with the occurrence of symptoms of depression as well as the risk of depressive illness. In most women, this is due to the psychological adjustments necessary after childbirth as well as to the loss of sleep and hard work entailed in caring for a baby.

Psychological mechanisms

The early psychoanalysts suggested that because the symptoms of depressive illness resemble those of mourning their causes may be similar. Thus, depression could be caused by loss of a loved one, a treasured object or pet, or a deeply felt ideal.

Most people regard gloomy thoughts as being secondary to depression. Recently, it has been proposed that such ideas ('depressive cognitions') may be the primary cause of depression, or they may aggravate and perpetuate the condition. Depressive cognitions can be divided into three types (see Table 4.2).

Any person who habitually falls into these ways of thinking will be more likely to become depressed over problems than a more optimistic person.

Table 4.2: *The three types of depressive cognitions.*

1	Thoughts,	e.g. 'I'm a failure as a parent.'
2	Expectations,	e.g. You cannot be happy unless everyone likes you
3	Distortions,	e.g. drawing conclusions without any evidence for them; concentrating on details and missing the important aspects of a situation; drawing a general conclusion on the basis of one incident; and relating events to oneself when it is unjustified

Conclusion

Little is known about the aetiology of depressive disorders, although there is evidence pointing to an important genetic component. The evidence indicates genetic heterogeneity and that there is no single aetiological basis for affective disorder. This would suggest that a classification based on clinical syndromes is unlikely to define aetiologically distinct subgroups of depression.

5 Suicide and Deliberate Self-harm

SUICIDE and deliberate self-harm (DSH) (parasuicide, attempted suicide) are overlapping behaviours. Their main characteristics are shown in Table 5.1.

Table 5.1: *Characteristics of suicide and deliberate self-harm.*

Suicide	Deliberate self-harm
Fatal	Non-fatal
Premeditated	Impulsive
Rates falling in recent years	Rates increasing in recent years
Rates increase with age	Rates decrease with age
More common in older males	More common in young females
Drugs and violence are common methods	Preponderance of drug overdose
Lower and upper social classes	Lower social class
Loss of parent by death in childhood	Broken home in childhood
Poor physical health	Good physical health
Normal premorbid personality	Abrupt mood swings or antisocial personality
70% have depression	10% have depression
Social isolation	Social disorganization

Adapted from Wilkinson (1989) *Depression* London: BMA.

Suicide

Suicide is an intentional act of self-destruction by a person cognisant of what he or she is doing and the probable consequences. Legally, there can be no presumption of suicide unless there is evidence of intention (e.g. a suicide note). The person must also have been capable of forming an intent.

Suicide in usually a feature of severe depressive illness but occasionally even mildly depressed patients succeed in killing themselves. Other factors are also important; suicide is more common in the elderly, the physically ill and in those who abuse alcohol, as well as in those who have made previous suicide attempts. About 15% of depressives eventually commit suicide.

Frequency

Official figures underestimate the incidence of suicide. Nevertheless, the suicide rate in the UK is one of the lowest in the world. Suicide is the sixth most frequent cause of death (after heart disease, cancer, respiratory disease, stroke and accidents), the third most common cause of death in the 15 – 44 year age-group, and it accounts for about 1 death every 3 – 4 years in a practice population of 2500.

Causes

Misfortune, mental illness and isolation from society are the main causes of suicide. Well-planned social and medical services are the means for recognizing and remedying them. Virtually all those who commit suicide (95%) are mentally ill before death: 70% are suffering from depression and 15% from alcoholism.

Medical contact

The majority of people who commit suicide have recently seen a doctor for treatment: 80% have seen their family doctor (75% in the month before suicide and 50% in the week before death); 25% have seen a psychiatrist (50% in the week before death); 80% have been prescribed psychotropic drugs.

Risk factors

The detection and improvement of risk factors (*see* Table 5.2) are vital. There is a particularly strong relationship between suicide and depressive illness.

Table 5.2: *Risk factors for suicide.*

Social	Illness	Symptoms
Male sex	Affective illness (particularly depression)	Suicidal thoughts
Age >45 years	Alcoholism and drug addiction	Severe depressed mood
Social classes V and I	Schizophrenia	Persistent insomnia

Table 5.2: *continued.*

Social	Illness	Symptoms
Separated, divorced or widowed status	Serious physical or chronic incapacitating illness	Marked loss of interest
Immigrant	Recent DSH (particularly using violent means)	Hopelessness
Social isolation	Personality disorder (mood antisocial)	Worthlessness and inadequacy
Unemployment and redundancy	Organic brain disease (early dementia, epilepsy, head injury)	Guilt and self-blame
Retirement	Family history of alcoholism	Agitation or retardation
Living in a socially disorganized area		Social withdrawal
Recent bereavement		Anger and resentment
Spring months		Unresolved or deteriorating health or social difficulties
		Self-neglect
		Memory impairment

Adapted from Wilkinson (1989) *Depression* London: BMA.

Deliberate self-harm

DSH, parasuicide and attempted suicide are non-fatal acts, most commonly involving the ingestion of substances (particularly psychotropic drugs) in excess of prescribed or recommended doses, but also including other types of self-injury. About 10% of episodes of DSH are failed suicides.

Frequency

There are over 100 000 cases of DSH in England and Wales annually. During 1 year, DSH will account for about 3 – 4 persons consulting in a practice population of 2500.

Management of Suicide

The repercussions of suicide affect close family and friends of the deceased as well as medical, nursing professionals and other people involved. Counselling, individual support and discussion within the practice may help relieve guilt and anger and prevent further complications.

Causes

The majority of patients inflicting DSH are not mentally ill. It is usually an impulsive response to a social crisis in a person whose vulnerability has been increased by alcohol. The main purpose of DSH is probably to communicate distress.

Patients inflicting DSH experience an increase in recent life-events, which is most marked in the preceding week (quarrels and arguments with a spouse or partner, family or friends; episodes of personal physical illness; examination crises; imminent court appearances; difficulties with children, finances, work, health and alcohol; a new person in the household; and family illness).

Medical contact

The majority of DSH patients seek medical help prior to the act: 65% have seen their GP in the month beforehand; 35% have seen their GP in the week beforehand; 20% have seen psychiatrists in the same time-intervals; 25% have seen a social worker, a member of the clergy or a voluntary agency in the month beforehand.

Assessment

A schematic guide to the assessment of patients after DSH is shown in Table 5.3, page 36.

Assessment of suicidal intent

About 1% of DSH patients commit suicide within 1 year of a previous DSH attempt and 10% commit suicide in the long term. The degree or nature of drug overdose or injury has no clear predictive value, and promises that suicidal impulses will not be acted upon are unreliable.

Table 5.3: *Assessment of patients after deliberate self-harm.*

Topic	Questions
The parasuicidal act	Circumstances Reasons, aims, expectations Premeditation Current suicidal intent Events in previous week Events in previous 24 hours
Current problems	Psychological Social Physical
Background factors	Previous DSH Personality Personal and family history
Current mental state	Depressive illness Schizophrenic illness Alcohol and/or drug abuse Cognitive function
Ability to cope	Previous methods of coping Current resources for coping

Finally it is important to establish what psychological, social and physical treatment is appropriate and/or acceptable to the patient now and in the future.

Particular significance should be attached to the presence of risk factors, mental illness (especially depressive illness), recent DSH (especially extensive laceration or jump from a height), precautions to prevent discovery, premeditation and absence of precipitating factors.

The patient should be asked sensitively about suicidal ideas and plans—contrary to popular belief there is no evidence that asking such questions 'plants a seed' in the patient's mind.

Suicidal thoughts are usually of slow onset, first appearing as a feeling that life is not worth living. Later, patients begin to think that it would be a relief to go to sleep and never wake up, or to die, or be killed suddenly. Preoccupations with death increase and become persistent; vague thoughts about suicide progress to possible methods and this culminates in a suicide attempt or suicide.

Use the following ascending hierarchy to assess suicidal intent.

- Does the patient feel life is not worth living?
- Does he or she wish to go to sleep and never wake up?
- Does he or she wish to die suddenly or be killed in an accident?
- Is there a preoccupation with death and dying?
- Are there vague thoughts of suicide?
- Do the patient's thoughts centre on methods of suicide?
- Has the patient plans to commit suicide?

Assessment of risk of repetition

About 15% of patients who have deliberately harmed themselves repeat the activity within 1 year. Repetition is strongly associated with:

- a previous episode;
- a history of psychiatric treatment;
- a criminal record;
- lower social class;
- separation from spouse/partner;
- an episode not precipitated by social crisis, drug dependence or alcoholism;
- early maternal separation.

Management of deliberate self-harm

The first priority is to ensure that the DSH patient's capacity for inflicting further self-harm is minimized, and that his or her medical condition is assessed and treated. A full psychosocial assessment should then be made.

The psychosocial assessment procedures have therapeutic potential. The majority of patients resolve family or personal problems around the time of DSH, either by themselves using their own resources or by using hospital/medical resources, or both, and by individual and joint counselling of all those involved. Doctors (with nurses and social workers) can facilitate the way the episode is resolved.

Virtually all patients should be admitted to a medical or DSH unit for appropriate medical treatment. Admission is normally overnight, or for 24 – 48 hours. Most patients who have inflicted DSH should be assessed by a psychiatrist after medical recovery and before discharge, although local policies do vary. Depending on clinical severity, patients found to have concurrent mental illness should be referred for specialist psychiatric assessment, preferably within 1 week of inflicting DSH.

Around 20% of patients who have deliberately harmed themselves require transfer to an inpatient psychiatric unit for detailed assessment and treatment. Rarely, a compulsory admission to a psychiatric hospital (under Section 2 of the Mental Health Act in England and Wales 1983) will be required, and this will usually be arranged with the co-operation of a psychiatrist.

Voluntary and social services agencies may be approached to provide support to socially disadvantaged patients. Despite all efforts, a large proportion of patients will default from whatever treatment is offered; in most cases, because the precipitating stress has been relieved. For this reason, the patient's preference for treatment should be considered in an attempt to ensure compliance.

Prevention of suicide and deliberate self-harm

Suicide is a major preventable cause of death, and DSH is one of the most easily identified risk factors for future suicide. **Remember:** at least 50% of those who commit suicide and DSH signal their intention to their doctor.

Primary prevention

The main primary prevention measures are: reduction in toxicity of domestic gas and drugs; improved management of DSH; improved assessment and treatment of mental illness; increased access to medical and social services; regular follow-up and social support for those at risk; care in prescribing psychotropic and other drugs to patients at risk, and to those who come into close contact with such patients; provision of information and advice to those at risk e.g. use of medical, social and voluntary services, vulnerability following alcohol, The Samaritans telephone counselling; improvement of the social and material circumstances of those at risk; reduction of the impact of risk factors; and the use of self-help groups.

Secondary and tertiary prevention

Unfortunately, no psychiatric or social intervention has been shown conclusively to prevent either suicide or the repetition of DSH. The main approaches are those mentioned above, but in particular depressive and other psychiatric (or physical) illnesses should be treated preferably by social and psychological means (including hospital treatment and regular follow-up) and with individual and family counselling rather than with psychotropic drugs, unless these are indicated clinically.

6 Professional Help

In a year, 3% of all of the hospital referrals made by an average GP are to specialist psychiatric clinics. The proportion of patients with mental health problems who are referred by GPs to psychiatrists and paramedical mental health workers *in general practice* is not known, but it is probably substantial.

There is also little information about the pattern of referrals for depression from GPs to psychiatrists and to paramedical providers of mental health care in general practice and how these relate to clinical outcome for patients. However, increasing numbers of patients are being referred in this way.

GPs and psychiatric outpatient clinics

It is intriguing to find that less than 50% of the patients attending psychiatric outpatient clinics need to remain under the direct supervision of consultants and even fewer require special facilities or treatments available only at hospital sites.

Fifty per cent of GPs use psychiatric outpatient clinics as a source of primary care or advice without first treating or investigating their patients, and psychiatrists tend to regard themselves as largely responsible for the total care of patients rather than as consultants. Consequently, there appears to be substantial blurring of the interface between primary and secondary psychiatric care, contributing in large measure to a mismatch between the observed and expected roles and functions of psychiatrists.

Th usual management decision made at initial specialist consultation is to continue outpatient treatment (the intended outcome for three-quarters of patients attending). Subsequently, however, about two-thirds of outpatients are seen on fewer than four occasions, and this rapid decline in attandance appears to be due equally to a high rate of discharge and of lapse from care.

For those attending more often, continuity of care tends to be unusual, with four-fifths of those attending on four or more occasions seeing different hospital doctors on different occasions. After 3 months, less than 50% of patients referred are still attending outpatients, 25% are receiving psychiatric treatment from their GP and around 25% are not receiving any treatment. Patients' clinical status at this time does not seem to be closely related to their treatment status, although those who decide to stop treatment tend to make relatively poor progress.

These observations may seem to reflect unfavourably on referral from GPs to psychiatrists. However, when asked, GPs indicate that in more than 50% of cases referral is helpful and that outcome broadly matches expectation, little or nothing is thought to have been achieved with 25% and, in a further 25%, the result is not known because the patient has not been seen again by the GP. Moreover, the attitudes of patients who attend outpatient clinics are also generally favourable to referral; their expectations of treatment tend to be low and in most cases realistic—a minority attend solely for social help.

Psychiatrists in primary care

About 1 in 5 consultant psychiatrists and psychotherapists in England and Wales (or their junior staff) spend roughly 1 session per week in general practice. Although few psychiatric attachments in general practice have been studied systematically, they are claimed to have important advantages over traditional outpatient clinics. For example, specialist psychiatric clinics in general practice appear to lead to an increase in the number of patients seen but a decrease in the number of new referrals seen in general practice; patients referred in the traditional way are more likely to have had previous contact with psychiatric services, to be admitted to hospital and to spend more time as inpatients.

Table 6.1: *Reasons for seeking advice from, or for referral to, a psychiatrist.*

- suicide risk;
- failure to eat or drink;
- treatment resistance;
- prevention of further episodes;
- specialized investigations;
- specialized treatment.

The psychiatrist usually treats patients who have the most severe depressive illnesses and those with particular associated medico-social difficulties. However, the majority of those referred to outpatients will receive only limited outpatient care. A minority may receive day- or inpatient care or at-home care.

In addition to the potent effects of the referral process, the psychiatrist can provide advice, information and help with more intensive general medical assessment and care, specialist drug treatment, electroconvulsive therapy (ECT) and access to a wider range of supportive/individual/group/marital/sexual/cognitive/behavioural/dynamic psychotherapies and social manipulations than a GP usually has.

Nurses

The role of nurses in the care of patients with depression and other forms of mental disorder has recently come under closer investigation, especially with the rapid, largely uncharted development of community psychiatric nursing services. In 1985, there were just under 3000 community psychiatric nurses (CPNs) in the UK; the projections are for 4500 by 1990, 7500 by 1995, and 12 500 by the year 2000.

Increases in numbers of this order suggest that radical changes in nursing practice will follow. It is worth noting that CPNs are tending increasingly to treat patients found in primary care rather than reducing demands made on traditional services.

GPs are the largest group of doctors referring patients to CPNs whether they are based in primary care or institutional settings. The most frequent reason for referral by GPs to CPNs working in health centres is for help in the treatment of patients with depression and anxiety.

It should also be noted that practice nurses already provide a great deal of emotional support to patients with depression and anxiety, although this is largely unrecognized and unrecorded. In addition, attention has recently been drawn to the important practical role of health visitors in identifying and treating emotional problems in postpartum women.

Social workers

Following a period of expansion in social services during the 1960s and 1970s, social services within the medical sector are now being retracted. There is some evidence that the more practical skills of social workers are useful in the management of chronic depression in general practice. The most likely explanation of the general benefits associated with a social work attachment in general practice is that the social worker's actions supplement the resources that she or he mobilizes, and facilitate a more positive approach by the GP towards the social orbit of morbidity.

The results of two randomized controlled trials have demonstrated the effectiveness of social work for depressed patients. In one study, women suffering from acute or acute-on-chronic depression were referred to a a social worker attached to a practice or for routine treatment by their GP. Women assessed initially as having acute-on-chronic depression with major marital difficulties were found to benefit from social work treatment. In the other study, depressed patients were allocated to individual cognitive therapy, group cognitive therapy or a waiting-list control group. Those who had cognitive therapy from a social worker did significantly better up to 1 year than those on the waiting list, but there was no significant difference between patients treated with group cognitive therapy and those treated with individual cognitive therapy.

Clinical psychologists

Around 14% of clinical psychologists work with GPs, and GPs refer to clinical psychologists patients who have a range of clinical difficulties, from anxiety, phobia, depression and psychosomatic conditions to habit disorders, behavioural, personality, interpersonal, social, marital, sexual, educational and occupational problems, and cognitive impairment.

The level of patient satisfaction with behavioural treatment is high, and patients have one-third to a half fewer consultations for advice or prescriptions for psychotropic medication in the year following psychological intervention. Such benefits have been confirmed up to 1 year in a randomized controlled clinical and economic evaluation of a behaviourally oriented clinical psychology service in a health centre. There is also evidence to suggest that contact with a psychologist may have effects on referred patients and their families in the longer term, with decreases at 3 years in psychotropic drug prescriptions for patients and in both consultations and prescriptions for their children.

Advantages have also been shown for specific psychological treatments in patients with depression. The results of 2 controlled clinical trials indicate that the use of cognitive therapy by psychologists in combination with antidepressants produces beneficial effects in the treatment of patients with depressive disorders.

Counselling

A growing number of counsellors are being recruited into primary care, where they are referred patients with anxiety, depression, the effects of acute or long-term stress, psychosomatic illness, marital problems and relationship difficulties, sexual problems, and difficulties arising subsequent to abortion or in relation to bereavement. Individual, family, group and marital counselling are used, and the counsellor's main aim is to offer the patient support and insight. Patients are also given the chance to learn new skills, such as relaxation, and vocational and educational guidance may be given. Several clinical accounts demonstrate the impact of counselling in general practice, for example, on the subjective feelings of patients and GPs, and in reducing the use of psychotropic drugs and the number of consultations.

People with marital difficulties are more likely to contact their GP for help than any other social service, and attachments of marriage guidance counsellors to practices have been set up to encourage GPs to refer patients directly. Although these attachments appear to work well, the experience is limited largely to self-selected and atypical practices.

Conclusion

Several controlled evaluations of specialist mental health treatment in primary care are now available. The main finding is that treatment by specialist mental health professionals is superior to usual GP treatment—the success rate of specialist treatment is just over 10% greater than that of usual GP treatment.

Counselling, behaviour therapy and general psychiatry prove to be similar in their overall effect. However, there is a degree of variability among different outcome categories. The influence of counselling seems to be greatest on social functioning, whereas behaviour therapy appears to exert its greatest impact on reducing contacts with outpatients.

Although most of the acutely ill patients with psychotic disorders see a psychiatrist, about 95% of patients with depressive illnesses (a greater problem from a public health point of view) are treated by GPs, usually entirely alone, but also sometimes in conjunction with various paramedical providers of mental health care.

Inasmuch as depression is a medical problem, GPs are the main providers of care, and the case for establishing general practice as the 'middle ground' for psychiatric treatment is strong. GPs become involved early in the detection and treatment of patients in the acute and chronic phases of depression, as well as when relapses occur; they provide a preventive framework, which recognizes the patient in the context of family and community, and continuity of mental health care; and they supply comprehensive general health care to a group of patients who tend to consult more often for physical illness. Another important factor is that the treatment of depression in general practice is less stigmatizing for the patients concerned.

In keeping with the current transition to the provision of more mental health care in the community and the greater availability of and access to paramedical workers, GPs seem to be turning increasingly to nurses, social workers, clinical psychologists and counsellors rather than to psychiatrists for additional help for their patients with depression. The available evidence supports the effectiveness of the different therapeutic approaches, although many more evaluative studies are required. Unfortunately many GPs have no alternative other than referral to a psychiatrist because no other service is available locally.

7 Medical Treatment

THERE are three principal modes of intervention available for people suffering from depressive illness: medical, psychological and social treatment. However, in practice, these elements tend to be combined in the various treatments offered by different professionals.

GPs, social workers, clinical psychologists, CPNs, counsellors and psychiatrists all have important roles to play in the treatment of people with depressive illness. Common to all their approaches and at least as important as the specific features of treatment are the general characteristics they display, i.e. acceptance, warmth, genuineness, empathy, a tolerant attitude, dependability, continuity and an interest that allows the professional to take even seemingly minor problems seriously.

Depressive illness is best treated by a combination of medical, psychological and social methods; associated physical illness also requires treatment.

The GP's role

The doctor's support, encouragement and explanations are powerful adjuncts to medical treatment, particularly when provided early and regularly. To begin with, the patient should be seen briefly at 2 – 3-day intervals and then weekly to ensure compliance, to monitor side-effects and to assess progress. A model for auditing the patient's progress and the process of care is described in the Appendix to this chapter (p. 65).

When embarking on the treatment of a patient with depression, it is important to bear in mind that most depressive illnesses remit within 3 – 12 months.

The elderly

In the management of elderly patients with depression, in addition to a full history, it is important to undertake a physical examination concentrating on the detection of cardiovascular disease, neoplasm, thyroid or vitamin B_{12} deficiency, electrolyte imbalance or early parkinsonism. A thorough check should be made of current medication. It is paticularly important to be aware of factors affecting altered drug response in elderly patients, *see* Table 7.1.

Table 7.1: *Factors affecting altered drug response in elderly patients.*

Altered function	Change	Effects
Bioavailability	↓ Gastrointestinal absorption	↓ drug in blood per unit of time
Distribution	↓ Plasma protein binding	↑ free drug available in blood
Metabolism	↓ Significant hepatic enzyme	Drug and metabolites active for ↑ duration
Body composition	↑ Ratio of fat to other tissue	↑ potential to store lipid-soluble drugs
Excretion	↓ Renal glomerular filtration and tubular secretion	↓ elimination of drugs
Receptors	↑ sensitivity	↑ dose response

Adapted from Derogatis and Wise (1989) *Anxiety and Depressive Disorders in the Medical Patient* Washington, DC: American Psychiatric Press, Inc.

Early action

The first step is to ensure the patient has a good night's sleep. An antidepressant drug with sedative properties may be prescribed. Sometimes this will cause excessive sedation on the first few nights, but it is usually best to start in this way and then reduce the dose gradually. Daytime restlessness or tension may also require antidepressant drug treatment, and the aim is to achieve relaxation without drowsiness.

Depressed people frequently feel lonely, and an attempt should be made to rally the support of family and friends because this usually helps. A temporary change of environment, such as going to stay with a friend or having a short holiday, may also bring relief.

In general, people suffering from depression who are still employed do not need to stop work or to break their social links. It is usually an advantage for the patient to keep occupied in these ways as they can help to improve self-esteem.

Advice and counselling

The GP should try to offer some simple counselling and advice to the patient. The following model could be used during the consultation.

Clarification of symptoms and problems. This includes encouraging the patient to talk about symptoms and contributing problems while asking questions to obtain a better understanding of the situation.

Explanation. Try to explain to the patient what is happening and how the symptoms have developed, e.g. the role of external stress or internal conflict via tensions in producing bodily symptoms.

Suggest ways of dealing with current problems. Involve the patient in the discussion. Encourage the patient to talk to his/her partner or other family members. Give advice regarding practical problems. Stress the need to come to terms with what cannot be changed (e.g. bereavement). Give basic advice regarding exercise, diet and leisure activities, and contact with other agencies – social services, Relate, Citizens' Advice Bureau, student counselling services, self-help groups (such as Cruse).

In milder cases it may be appropriate to give arguments against prescribing drugs: the patient's own coping resources should be sufficient to deal with the problems; the problems the patient faces are 'life problems' rather than an illness or a medical condition; drugs mask the symptoms but do not treat the original causes; drugs also have side-effects.

Further appointments. Convey a willingness to discuss the problems again if the patient wants to, and make a definite arrangement for a further appointment.

These measures alone may lead to a general lifting of depression, and acute depression triggered by life-events and mild – moderate depression may improve within a few days of early medical treatment.

Specific treatment

If such depressions do not lift, or if any improvement is only temporary (7 – 14 days' duration), more specific treatment is required.

For more seriously depressed people, referral to a psychiatrist for out- or day-patient care, even admission to hospital, may have to be considered at the outset, particularly if there is:

- immediate risk of suicide or DSH;
- risk of harm being caused to others;
- antisocial behaviour;
- a particularly unhelpful home environment.

In these situations, compulsory admission to hospital may be life-saving.

Medical management of depressive illness

The main medical treatment for patients who have depressive illness is antidepressant drugs. ECT is sometimes helpful for those with severe illness. Psychosurgery is rarely used but has a place in the management of severe intractable depressive illness.

The results of many randomized controlled clinical trials in both general and specialist practice attest to the superiority of antidepressant drugs over placebo. However, remember that:

- no patient is adequately treated with *antidepressant drugs* alone;
- *counselling* might be particularly useful when depression seems to arise from the effects of early deprivation;
- an unrewarding lifestyle suggests the need for *social and behavioural changes*;
- pronounced negative thinking suggests that a *cognitive approach* may be helpful;
- *ECT* is safe and effective in treating more serious depressive illnesses, where there is a strong risk of suicide or when a quick response is essential because the depression is life-threatening.

Antidepressant drugs

Indications

The main indications for antidepressant drugs are to relieve symptoms; to help shorten the length of an episode of depression; to provide maintenance treatment against relapse.

Antidepressant drugs are particularly indicated when a diagnosis of moderate-to-severe depression is made and the following symptoms are present:

- sleep disturbance;
- loss of appetite;
- loss of weight;
- loss of libido;
- loss of interests;
- inactivity;
- fatigue;
- marked anxiety;
- impaired concentration;
- suicidal thoughts;
- agitation or retardation.

The presence of a number of these symptoms in association with depression is a useful measure of the patient's 'psychobiological response'; the more pronounced this response is, the more likely it is that antidepressant drugs will help.

The presence of stress is of little relevance to the use of anti-depressants. It is best to ignore presumed causes and focus on the pattern of symptoms. Thus, treatment may be expected to affect depressive symptoms but not an unhappy development or an unrewarding lifestyle.

First choice antidepressant drugs

Tricyclic (or related) antidepressants are first-line drugs. The two longest established and best known are amitriptyline (which is more sedative—agitated and anxious patients benefit more) and imipramine (which is less sedative than amitriptyline—withdrawn, apathetic or retarded patients benefit more).

Mechanism of action

Clinical manifestations of depressive illness may be associated with a deficiency of noradrenaline and serotonin at central neuronal synapses in the brain. Monoamine deficiency may be corrected by antidepressant drugs whose primary pharmacological action is to inhibit the re-uptake of noradrenaline and serotonin by the presynaptic nerve terminals within the brain, thus increasing transmitter levels at central synapses and so producing behavioural stimulation and a clinical antidepressant effect.

The monoamine deficiency hypothesis does not fully account for the mechanism of action of antidepressants, especially the latency of their clinical effect. In depressive illness, it is believed that the brain is in a state of noradrenergic supersensitivity and that normal or subnormal amounts of released noradrenaline are insufficient to maintain regular neurotransmission. Cortical noradrenaline receptor density and noradrenaline stimulated cyclic-AMP production are parameters that reflect the regulatory state.

Dose Build up from 75 to 225 mg/day depending on the development of side-effects.

Delay in action The antidepressant effects may take 2 – 3 weeks to become apparent.

Maintenance treatment

Maintaining treatment for 6 – 9 months after response to an antidepressant may halve the relapse rate.

- Prescribe a limited supply at first because of the possibility of suicidal tendencies developing just at the time when the patient is improving and becoming more active.
- Low doses should be used initially in the elderly.
- If doses up to 225 mg/day for 1 month fail to produce a response, it is unlikely that another tricyclic antidepressant will be effective.

Indications for alternative antidepressant drug treatment

The main indications for alternative antidepressant drug treatment are:

- side-effects of first choice treatments;
- no response to first choice treatments;

- medical illnesses incompatible with the first choice
  treatments, e.g. mianserin, iprindole and doxepin may
  be preferred if cardiotoxicity is a problem.

Alternative antidepressant drugs

- Those with more sedative effects: dothiepin, doxepin,
  maprotiline, mianserin, trazodone, trimipramine.
- Those with less sedative effects: butriptyline, clomipramine,
  desipramine, imipramine, iprindole, lofepramine,
  nortriptyline, viloxazine.
- Those with stimulant action: protriptyline.

Compliance

Compliance with the prescription of antidepressant drugs is probably quite low: there is a 20 – 60% treatment drop-out rate at 3 weeks. Therefore, attempts to improve compliance are particularly important.

The largest group of non-compliers (30 – 40%) stop taking antidepressant drugs because of the expectation or presence of side-effects. Expectation may be a powerful demotivating force.

In patients who experience side-effects on antidepressant drugs, the most common reason for stopping medication is a dry mouth, which is very poorly tolerated.

1 *Advise the patient.* In the first few days, antidepressants help most with any sleep problems and tend to have a calming effect, sometimes making people feel more lethargic. However, this effect gives way to increasing alertness and energy after 1 – 2 weeks of regular medication. Later it may be important to advise the patient that:

- immediate benefits from antidepressants should not be
  expected; it may take 4 – 6 weeks before the maximum
  benefit of antidepressant medication is apparent;
- antidepressant treatment will usually need to continue until
  symptoms disappear;
- after 1 month of wellbeing, the dose of antidepressant may
  slowly be reduced, continuing for 1 – 2 weeks at each new
  dose level, guarding lest symptoms reappear, which is likely
  if drug withdrawal is premature;

- some patients benefit from maintenance antidepressant treatment at a lower dose for about 6 – 9 months to prevent relapse;
- antidepressant treatment is usually reduced when social circumstances are stable;
- antidepressant treatment should probably not be reduced if special life stresses arise.

2 *Side-effects of antidepressant drugs.* Patients should be warned of likely side-effects. These are common, and at their worst in the first few days of starting or of increasing the dose, but they are usually mild and reversible. Older people may be especially sensitive to side-effects, particularly dizziness and fainting. Patients should be advised to record and report side-effects to the doctor, for advice on what to do.

In most cases, the antidepressant dose may be taken 2 – 3 hours before bedtime so that the patient is asleep when he or she might otherwise be troubled by side-effects, or the prescription may be changed to an antidepressant lacking the particular side-effect that the patient has suffered.

Side-effects

The following side-effects may occur within a day of starting antidepressant drugs:

- dry mouth;
- blurring of vision;
- postural hypotension;
- ventricular tachycardias and ECG changes;
- tachycardia;
- sweating;
- constipation;
- headache;
- difficulty passing urine;
- confusion;
- sedation, drowsiness and unsteadiness e.g. with amitriptyline;
- rarely alertness e.g. with nortriptyline.

Most of these side-effects usually respond to a reduced dose or change in medication.

Later side-effects, i.e. those that occur 2 or more weeks after medication has commenced, include:

- tremor;
- weight gain;
- disturbed sexual function.

These usually recede with a reduced dose, or a change in drug.

Neurological, dermatological, haematological and hepatic side-effects have also been reported.

It is also important to tell the patient to avoid driving (until used to the drug) and alcohol whilst taking medication.

Special precautions with tricyclic antidepressants are required in patients with:

- prostatic conditions causing urinary retention;
- glaucoma;
- cardiovascular disease;
- epilepsy;
- diabetes mellitus;
- hyperthyroidism;
- hypertension;
- liver disorders;
- psychoses;
- suicidal tendencies.

Tricyclic antidepressants are contraindicated in patients with:

- acute myocardial infarction;
- heart block;
- pregnancy;
- severe liver disease.

It should be borne in mind that in most antidepressant drug trials many unwanted effects are reported both before response and during the continuation phase of treatment. However, the incidence of most unwanted effects is as high among patients receiving placebo and so the presence of side-effects cannot be attributed directly to the active drug. The main exception is a dry mouth which may occur more frequently in those who continue with treatment but who have previously noted this effect.

Hints for patients and GPs on dealing with adverse effects

Atropine-like side-effects

- Dry mouth: suggest regular sips of water or fruit/sweets/chewing gum.
- Constipation: suggest high-fibre diet—green vegetables, bran, etc.—and adequate fluid intake.

In general, these effects are short-lived and entirely reversible. They may lessen or disappear within the first 2 – 3 days of starting a standard tricyclic antidepressant.

If such effects are persistent or intolerable, reduce the dose by 25 mg (or more, depending on severity) of a standard tricyclic antidepressant at intervals of 3 – 4 days until they are no longer troublesome.

Other adverse effects

- Drowsiness, if mild, may be welcomed initially by some patients.
- Postural hypotension: warn against rising quickly from chair, bed or bath.

With these adverse effects, it will usually be necessary to reduce the dose of standard tricyclic antidepressant by 25 mg (or more depending on severity) at intervals of 3 – 4 days.

Thorough medical assessment

The occurrence of tachycardia, postural hypotension or rash will usually warrant a thorough medical assessment. *See* Table 7.2 for important interactions between tricyclic antidepressants and other drugs.

Lack of response

Patients with depressive illnesses occasionally do not respond to tricyclic or related antidepressants. In these circumstances review:

- diagnosis;
- patient's treatment compliance;
- any unresolved life difficulties.

Table 7.2: *Interactions between tricyclics and other drugs.*

Drug	Nature of interaction
Alcohol	CNS depression, ↓ reaction time
α-Adrenergic agonists	↑ of the agonist
Amphetamines	↑ tricyclic effects; hypertension, arrhythmia
Anticholinergics	Toxic delirium, confusion, visual hallucinations
Anticoagulants (oral)	↑ anticoagulant effects
Anticonvulsants	↓ of the seizure threshold
Antihistamines	Enhanced anticholinergic effects
Antihypertensives	Antagonism of antihypertensive action in some drugs; enhancement of hypotensive effects in others
Antipsychotics	↑ tricyclic blood levels
Anxiolytics	↑ sedation
Ascorbic acid	↑ excretion of tricyclics
Barbiturates	↑ sedation; ↓ tricyclic blood levels through ↑ metabolism
β-Adrenergic blockers	Antagonism of blocker action
Cimetidine	↑ tricyclic effects and blood levels
Digitalis	Possible enhancement of digitalis
Monoamine oxidase inhibitors	↑ of antidepressant effect; hypotensive or hypertensive crisis; hyperpyrexia; convulsions
Narcotics	Mutual enhancement
Quinidine	↑ quinidine effects
Sympathomimetics	↑ sympathomimetic effects
Thyroid hormones	↑ antidepressant effects; possible ↑ thyroid effect

Adapted from Derogatis and Wise (1989) *Anxiety and Depressive Disorders in the Medical Patient* Washington, DC: American Psychiatric Press, Inc.

If these enquiries are unproductive, supportive and antidepressant treatment should continue as outlined above, bearing in mind the likelihood of remission between 3 and 12 months.

The temptation to overtreat should be resisted. In exceptional circumstances, other types of antidepressant drugs may be tried (see below), either alone or in combination. These treatments can cause medical difficulties and are best prescribed with specialist advice. The chief examples are:

- monoamine oxidase inhibitors (MAOIs);
- flupenthixol (low dose);
- tryptophan;
- carbamazepine;
- lithium.

Monoamine oxidase inhibitors

MAOIs are used infrequently because of the dangers of serious dietary and drug interactions. The main examples are:

- phenelzine;
- isocarboxazid;
- tranylcypromine (most hazardous because of stimulant action).

Depressed patients with anxieties, phobias and bodily symptoms, and those who have failed to respond to tricyclic or related antidepressants sometimes respond well to treatment with MAOIs.

As the response to MAOIs may take 3 weeks or more to become apparent, it is necessary to give them for a trial period lasting about 4 – 6 weeks before concluding that they are ineffective.

Interactions with monoamine oxidase inhibitors   Certain drugs and tyramine-containing foods cause an interaction with MAOIs leading to a dangerous rise in blood pressure—an early warning of which is a throbbing headache. This interaction lasts for up to 14 days after treatment with MAOIs has ceased.

Tricyclic and relation antidepressants should not be taken until at least 14 days after MAOI treatment has been stopped.

What to advise the patient   While taking MAOIs and for up to 14 days after stopping such treatment:

- do not eat cheese, pickled herring or broad bean pods;
- do not eat or drink Bovril, Oxo, Marmite, or similar meat or yeast extract;

- eat only fresh foods, and avoid game and any food that could be stale or 'going off', especially meat, fish, poultry or offal;
- do not take any other medicines (including treatment for coughs and colds, pain relievers, tonics and laxatives) without consulting your doctor or pharmacist, whether these were purchased over the counter or prescribed by your doctor;
- avoid alcoholic drinks;
- record and report any unusual or severe symptoms to your GP.

Side-effects

- dizziness;
- insomnia;
- increased appetite;
- agitated feeling;
- otherwise similar to other antidepressants (*see* p. 53).

Other drugs sometimes used in the treatment of depression

Various other drugs may be useful for some of the symptoms of depression. Tranquillizers, such as diazepam or thioridazine, are sometimes given, particularly if worry and agitation are severe. Unfortunately, these drugs may slow down patients' thinking and further reduce their energy levels and therefore they are probably best used only in exceptional cases.

Lithium

Lithium salts are sometimes used in the prevention or limitation of depressive illnesses, as well as in the treatment of manic episodes. Suitable patients have to be selected carefully and treatment is usually carried out under specialist guidance. As lithium is prescribed for relatively long periods (3 – 5 years initially, and sometimes 'for life'), the likelihood of recurrence of depression has to be weighed against the risks and side-effects of the treatment, which in this case are greater than usual and require very careful monitoring, including 3 monthly blood tests and medical examinations to ensure that the level of lithium in the blood is stable within a narrow range.

Side-effects

The main side-effects of lithium are due to high blood lithium levels, sometimes aggravated by the use of diuretics or dehydration. The signs of lithium toxicity are progressive and include:

- tremor;
- blurred vision;
- passing excess urine;
- thirst leading to drinking excessive fluids;
- anorexia, vomiting and diarrhoea;
- mild drowsiness and sluggishness;
- giddiness and incoordination;
- slurring;
- eye problems;
- kidney problems;
- seizures.

Most of these side-effects are reversed when the dose is reduced or the drug temporarily stopped. Patients should be warned to ask the doctor for advice if such side-effects persist or seem to be progressing because eventually loss of consciousness can occur if no action is taken to reduce the blood lithium level.

Long-term use of lithium may be associated with changes in kidney tissue and function, and thyroid, skin and heart problems—further important reasons why the decision to use lithium has to be weighed carefully against the severity of the depressive illness and the potential it may have for disrupting the patient's life and work.

Electroconvulsive therapy

ECT is mainly used to treat patients with severe and life-threatening depressive illnesses, particularly if patients have stopped eating and drinking because of their illness, or if they have acute delusions or other psychotic symptoms, or strong suicidal ideas and urges. In all these circumstances, a quick and sure response is required. ECT is usually also considered for people who remain severely depressed after antidepressant drug treatment, and other methods have failed to produce the desired response.

What to advise the patient

ECT involves having a small current of electricity passed through the brain via both temples (bilateral ECT) or via one temple (unilateral ECT) while the patient is under a general anaesthetic. The treatment is usually carried out for patients who are already in hospital, but occasionally ECT is given to outpatients. Although the procedure is safe, painless and without many side-effects, it has a frightening and offputting image.

ECT causes the patient to have a mild convulsion. The mechanism of action is not known, but it is thought that ECT influences the chemical transmitter systems in the brain.

Within a few minutes of administering ECT, the anaesthetic wears off and the patient comes round. Sometimes the patient experiences mild confusion, headache, stiff muscles or nausea for an hour or so, but with rest these effects pass off uneventfully.

ECT is the quickest treatment for the more severe types of depressive illness, and patients receiving ECT begin to show improvement within days or a week of commencing therapy. The treatment is given as a course, usually 6 sessions of ECT at a rate of 2 per week. Some people benefit from longer courses or from more frequent applications, depending on individual circumstances and responses.

It is safe to perform ECT in the frail, the elderly, those with high blood pressure, those with Parkinson's disease, those who have heart problems or who have sustained a stroke (from about 3 months after an attack) and in pregnancy. The risks of ECT are equivalent to those involved in having a general anaesthetic for other reasons.

Memory impairment?

One of the most common complaints made of ECT is that it causes memory impairment, for example, patients have difficult in remembering names or learning new information. This is particularly likely to happen in older people who have depression and accompanying dementing illness. In fact, although a great deal of research has been done to try and identify exactly what the memory problems are, conflicting results have been obtained and there is no definite evidence that ECT causes memory disturbance.

Such complaints are made less frequently of unilateral ECT, which is usually given on the right temple (in right-handed people) to avoid affecting the speech centre of the brain, disturbance of which is thought to be responsible for confusion and memory complaints. Such difficulties, when they do arise, are usually short-lived, disappearing within a few weeks of stopping treatment.

In common with all treatments, the patient has the right to refuse consent for ECT. Although with respect to drugs if a patient accepts a prescription he or she is deemed to be consenting to treatment, in the case of ECT a patient is asked to sign a consent form before treatment can be given.

Relapse prevention

Prevention of depression using antidepressant drugs

Patients with frequent recurrences of depressive illness or chronic depression are sometimes maintained on antidepressants for periods of several years in an effort to prevent or 'damp down' future episodes. This seems to be a safe procedure if it is undertaken under medical supervision. However, regular consideration should always be given to the continuing need for long-term antidepressant medication.

After recovery, the patient should be seen regularly, e.g. monthly, for several months. It should be made clear to the patient that he or she can be seen earlier than the next appointment if necessary.

If recovery appears to be associated with the use of antidepressants, patients should be continued at about half the previous dose or above for a period of around 6 months, because this may halve the relapse rate.

Indications of relapse are a return of depressive symptoms. It may be helpful to ask the patient and relatives to report signs of illness returning. Adjustments to lifestyle and personal attitudes that may have contributed to the onset or persistence of depression may be started at this stage.

Prevention of recurrent depression and manic illness

Lithium salts (see p. 58) are sometime used in the prevention or limitation of recurrent depressive illnesses, particularly when associated with manic episodes. Treatment of these patients is best carried out under specialist guidance.

Refractory depression

Refractory depression occurs when a patient's depressive illness is not responsive to an adequate course of treatment with an appropriate antidepressant of proven effectiveness (e.g. amitriptyline given in a dose of 150 mg for at least 6 weeks).

Most patients recover within 6 months. Those failing to respond tend to be referred to psychiatrists, often presenting with co-existing medical conditions, intractable social problems and severe personality difficulties.

Compliance

Poor treatment compliance is among the most common causes of treatment failure. Between 25 and 50% of patients fail to comply with treatment, the most common error being irregular and insufficient dosing. Complex dose schedules are less likely to be adhered to than simple once-nightly schedules. Early adverse drug effects often cause the patient to stop taking the drugs. Thus, provision of adequate information and explanation about side-effects is necessary at the time of prescription.

Non-compliance is common and remediable. It should be suspected in every case of treatment failure.

Organic causes of chronic depression

Treatment failure should lead to a review of the patient's history and clinical state for organic factors that may be perpetuating the condition. Infectious mononucleosis, hepatitis, viral pneumona and brucellosis are associated with depressive symptoms either during the acute illness or during a protracted recovery phase. Malignancies, particularly pancreatic cancer, should also be considered. Endocrine disturbances are also frequencly associated with depression. Addison's disease, Cushing's syndrome, hypothyroidism, hyperthyroidism, hyperparathyroidism and poorly controlled diabetes mellitus may all perpetuate depressive symptoms.

Early dementia is difficult to distinguish from depression in the elderly. Epilepsy, especially temporal lobe epilepsy, is associated with complex affective states. Cerebral tumours may present as depressive illnesses. Parkinsonism is associated with chronic depression which may be overlooked because of the other features of the disorder. Occasionally, multiple sclerosis and any chronic neurological disorder, is complicated by depression.

Several drugs are associated with depression, e.g. antihypertensive agents, such as reserpine and methyldopa, corticosteroids and oral contraceptives, centrally active substances such as barbiturates, antipsychotics, amphetamines and appetite suppressants, and narcotics, such as cocaine and heroin. Signs of alcohol dependence should also be sought.

Psychosocial factors

It may be useful to interview an informant about the patient's previous personality and present circumstances. Depressive personalities tend to be resistant to antidepressant drugs.

Exploring the symbolic significance of a seemingly trivial event may sometimes be productive. Events involving loss are particularly important. Key areas are the home, the family, the work place and leisure activities.

Pharmacokinetics

There are important individual variabilities in drug metabolism, and plasma levels of nortriptyline and amitriptyline should be monitored if facilities are available. The most important drug interaction involving tricyclic antidepressants is that with barbiturates. Barbiturates accelerate the metabolism of many tricyclic antidepressants thereby negating their effects. In contrast, phenothiazines compete for the drug metabolizing enzymes in the liver so that plasma concentrations of both drugs are elevated.

Clinical assessment of patients' antidepressant drug compliance

Ask the patient about autonomic side-effects. Persistent constipation, dry mouth and blurring of vision imply high serum concentrations. The 'near point' of vision steadily recedes as drug concentrations increase. This strategy is not helpful with newer antidepressants, such as mianserin, which have few anticholinergic effects.

Another strategy is to increase drug dose by stepwise gradual increments until the side-effects become apparent and then to decrease the dose by 1 unit (25 mg of a tricyclic antidepressant). Similarly, if side-effects are present without therapeutic benefit, the dose may be slowly decreased.

Alternative treatments

Alternative treatments include ECT, MAOIs, a combination of tricyclic antidepressants and MAOIs, tetracyclic antidepressants and other newer antidepressants, antipsychotic drugs, tryptophan and psychosurgery. Such treatments usually require specialist psychiatric management.

Five to 15% of depressed patients seem to be refractory to all forms of treatment. Most will eventually remit spontaneously, but a minority become chronic. Such patients require regular medical attention and support as well as carefully considered regular therapeutic initiatives.

Appendix: *Depression Audit*

Burton and Freeling reported a simple practical model for auditing management of depressive illness in primary care (*Journal of the Royal College of General Practitioners*, 1982; 32, 558 – 561). A modification of their basic scheme is outlined below, and can easily be adapted further, using more headings, for use in GP files. It is intended that a standardized record is kept of each depressed patient's condition at each consultation so that the patient's progress and the process of care can be assessed more reliably.

Assessment of depressive episode

	Very severe	Severe	Moderate	Mild	Not at all
Verbal report					
Behaviour					
Secondary symptoms					

Verbal report includes: unhappiness; worthlessness, helplessness, hopelessness; loss of interest; reported crying; death wishes.

Behaviour includes: looking sad; characteristic hunched depressed posture; tearfulness; sad, monotonous voice; slow movement.

Secondary symptoms include: insomnia; constipation; vague aches and pains; recent deliberate self-harm; loss of appetite and weight (both may rarely increase); difficulty concentrating or remembering.

Current impact of life-events

Contributing physical conditions

Drug(s)

Dosage schedule: Quantity
                                              prescribed:

Advice, information and help provided
Action/activity suggested
Side-effects
Compliance
Next appointment

8 Psychological Treatment

The traditional medical approach to the treatment of depression has been criticized for having a limited outlook and for neglecting personal and social issues. As a result, a variety of specialist psychological treatment approaches have been developed to treat depression (particularly mild depression), either as an adjunct to medical treatment or independently. Psychological treatments may be of value in mild – moderate depressive illness and may also have a beneficial role in the long-term treatment of those with severe depressive illness.

Although these treatments could be administered by a trained GP, most practitioners do not have the necessary time available and specialist referral is necessary. In mild depression and with intelligent patients, it may be possible to achieve considerable benefit by simply outlining the main principles to the patient.

Psychotherapy

Basis of psychotherapy

Any treatment for depression that does not include the prescription of drugs or other physical methods could be termed psychotherapy. The main component in all psychotherapies is talking, and it is the way in which words are used and the nature of the relationships formed between patients and therapists that differentiate the various forms of psychotherapy.

At first, many depressed patients seem unable to express anger or hostility. One psychotherapeutic view of depression is that it is inward turning of the aggressive instinct. Freud emphasized the significance of loss (of loved ones, objects or cherished ideas) in depression, drawing attention to the similarities between mourning and melancholia.

Other schools propose that humans have an innate tendency to seek attachments that lead to reciprocal, personal, social bonds with significant others and experiences of warmth, nurture and protection. Disruption of these bonds may then render individuals vulnerable to depression.

In psychotherapy, on the basis of such observations, the patient may be aided in attempting to redirect his or her hostility at more appropriate external objects, or the patient may be helped to examine current personal relationships and to understand how they have developed from experiences with attachment figures in childhood, adolescence and adulthood. The concept of attachment bonds provides a basis for understanding the personal background of depression and for developing strategies to correct distortions produced by faulty attachments in childhood. The value of strong attachment bonds appears to be especially great when individuals are faced with adversity.

Evidence to support the importance of interpersonal and social bonds is derived from the observation that people with depression tend to have fewer good friends and fewer contacts outside the household.

Psychotherapeutic approach

The psychotherapeutic approach in the treatment of depression has arisen from such theories as are outlined above. Disturbances in personal relationships are viewed as antecedents to depression and it is assumed that a depressed mood arises from relationship difficulties, e.g.:

- loss;
- disputes about roles (especially of the roles of husband and wife);
- role transitions (becoming a mother, a divorcee);
- lack of close relationships.

Psychotherapists therefore focus on:

- current and past relationships with significant people, such as the patient's family and friends;
- the quality and pattern of these relationships, with respect to:

  i   dealing with authority figures;
  ii dealing with dominance and submission;
  iii dependence and autonomy;
  iv intimacy, trust and sexual relationships;

- responses to separation and loss.

The concerns in psychotherapeutic treatment are to identify problems in a patient's closest relationships, and to consider with him or her alternative ways of behaving and thinking. The discussions between the patient and therapist concentrate on:

- emotions generated by close relationships (including warmth, anger, trust, envy and jealousy);
- family;
- friendship;
- work;
- attitudes to neighbourhood and community.

However, such treatment, especially in the form of psychoanalysis, is often prolonged, intensive and expensive. In addition, it is not readily available, and it is very difficult to assess its benefits. This applies to psychotherapy given individually or in groups. For these reasons, and because it is possible for patients to feel worse after psychotherapy, it is generally considered to be an inappropriate treatment for the majority of patients with depressive illness.

Support and counselling

GPs and most health professionals frequently find themselves in the position of giving emotional support, advice and counselling to depressed patients in an effort to provide reassurance, encouragement and sympathy. Indeed, this is probably the most common and most successful treatment for the bulk of patients with mild and moderate depressive illnesses. In this siutation, listening may be more important than giving advice, provided that listening means not only hearing the words spoken but also attending to what the patient is saying and trying to understand how he or she feels.

The main factors involved in support and counselling are as follows.

1 Expressing emotions appropriate to the situation:

- being reassured of the normality of emotions;
- a hand on the shoulder or having a tissue for tears may do more good than any number of words;
- irrational anger and guilt accepted by others.

2   Talking through events leading up to the crisis:

- to test the reality of events described;
- to explore the implications.

3   Encouragement to seek new directions in life:

- beware of seeing problems as entirely due to sickness;
- beware of becoming dependent on professional helpers.

It should not be forgotten that much of this support and counselling of people with depression is provided by ministers of religion, and voluntary bodies, most notably The Samaritans.

Cognitive therapy

Cognitive therapy is a relatively new form of psychological treatment in which it is proposed that a style of thinking characterized by negative expectations is the basis of depressive moods. Hopelessness and helplessness are central features of depression and reflect a 'cognitive triad' of a negative conception of the self, negative interpretations of one's experiences and a negative view of the future.

According to this theory there are two types of abnormality in depression.

1   Intrusive thoughts concerned with low self-regard, self-criticism and self-blame are common.

2   Cognitive distortions are also present which bias the patient's view of reality and make it possible for him or her to believe in the ideas represented in the intrusive thoughts.

Four kinds of cognitive distortions are described:

1   forming an interpretation when there is no factual evidence to support the conclusions or when the conclusion is contrary to evidence;

2   focusing on a detail taken out of context and ignoring other salient features;

3   drawing conclusions on the basis of a single incident;

4   magnification or minimization of errors when evaluating situations.

The cognitive approach centres on the notion that the way we think affects our emotions and behaviour. This explanation of depression can be contrasted with the traditional view which regards cognitive dysfunction as a symptom of depression rather than its cause. For instance, the mood swings which are a typical feature of depression are brought on by the patient's own thoughts. These take the form of negative ideas concerning the person in relation to his or her environment which have been rehearsed over a number of years. As with many bad habits, the individual is generally unaware of what he or she is doing.

The aims of cognitive therapy are to help the patient to recognize unhelpful automatic thoughts and then replace them with more flexible and adaptive cognitive responses. Cognitive techniques used in the treatment of depressive disorders attempt to alter maladaptive thinking by using verbal techniques, including explanation, discussion and questioning of assumptions, as follows.

1 *Identify recurrent intrusive thoughts* that increase depressed mood, by getting the patient to keep written records of moods and thinking in everyday life.

2 *Counterbalance negative thinking* by getting the patient to examine the evidence for and against these ideas and in doing so, to become aware of and correct the logical errors that allow him or her to arrive at and sustain these erroneously negative ideas and beliefs. The aim is to help the patient challenge the underlying assumptions and to find appropriate alternative ideas.

3 *Problem-solving* by helping patients to work out solutions to persistent life problems that help to maintain depression:

- define the problem;
- divide it into manageable parts;
- think of alternative solutions;
- select the best solution;
- carry it out and examine the result.

4 *Change the patient's behaviour* by helping the patient choose actions that are likely to change negative ways of thinking, i.e. 'learning from experience'. Some therapists recommend methods of increasing patients' assertiveness; others use 'pleasant event therapy', which focuses on increasing the patient's pleasant and rewarding experiences; and some employ 'self-control therapy', which emphasizes self-monitoring, self-evaluation and

self-reinforcement to correct problems with self-control in relation to coping with negative experiences.

If an individual distorts the evidence in one or more of these ways, 'automatic' depressive thoughts are likely to be unrealistic and maladaptive. It is not sufficient to help the patient modify the content of a particular thought and it is essential that he or she should come to recognize and modify the reasoning process that led to a false conclusion if similar errors are to be avoided in the future.

Although the cognitive therapist pays particular attention to the 'automatic' thoughts that precede a change of mood, he or she is also concerned with questioning the deeper assumptions an individual makes about the world, because the deeper assumptions provide the 'automatic' thought with power.

Management

First step

The first step is to help the patient to become aware of such negative thinking and to recognize the relationship between it and depressive changes of mood. This can be done by helping an individual to recognize 'automatic' thoughts during treatment, when the depressive episode can be relived using role play.

Second step

The second step is to help the patient to develop different ways of interpreting events; for example, an individual may be encouraged to stand back from a problem in order to get a more objective view. Different ideas may be sought and the patient asked to rate their correctness.

Once the patient is generating alternatives in interpreting events, he or she may be asked to keep a daily record of mood changes and the thoughts associated with them. The individual may be asked to reason with 'automatic' thoughts and suggest other possible interpretations to him- or herself as soon as a lowering of mood becomes apparent.

Third step

The third step of the process is to encourage the patient to test out beliefs and attitudes associated with depression in a systematic way. Instead of treating ideas as fact, the patient is helped to see that it is possible to discover the truth or otherwise of his or her beliefs through inquiry.

Progression

Progressively, treatment prepares the patient for change, but usually a change in behaviour is required before most are willing to discard a false belief altogether. One way to bring this about is for the therapist and patient to identify a relevant task that the patient can carry out as 'homework'.

As the patient improves and learns the cognitive approach, the focus of treatment moves to the deeper assumptions believed to underly the individual's depressive thinking. Unless these are identified and modified, the patient is likely to become depressed again in the future. As these beliefs have usually been present from an early age they are highly resistant to change. There are no simple techniques for eliciting such assumptions. A useful start is for the patient to identify recurring depressive themes in his or her life. The best way to break the pattern is to encourage the patient to act against these deeper assumptions.

Psychologists have found that most patients with depression respond to 15 – 30 sessions over 3 months, i.e. their depression is 'cured' or lifts. Two sessions a week are usually held in the first month, followed by weekly meetings thereafter.

9 Social Treatment

For the sociologist, depression is the outcome of a social structure that deprives individuals, with certain roles in life, of control of their destiny. This view focuses on processes such as urbanization, the influence of social class, racial membership, ethnic background and political and economic forces in the causation of depression and provides an explanation for increased rates of mental illness among certain groups, such as the increased rates of depression among working class women. As an example, a feminist interpretation of the high rates of depression in women would be that women are oppressed and that depressive feelings of helplessness and worthlessness are understandable in terms of womens' current status in society.

Practice

In practical terms, social treatment covers all efforts to improve a patient's well-being by altering aspects of his or her social life, particularly in relation to family relationships, work and leisure activities. Of course, defined in this way, virtually all treatment consists of some social elements (even visiting the GP is a social event).

At the most simple level, having a holiday, taking time off work or taking up a new interest are all important social means of trying to relieve depression. Family and voluntary social support can take the form of visiting and/or befriending depressed people—this can bring relief to the depressed person through the presence of a sympathetic ear and shoulder to cry on. Education and religion also offer great opportunities for social sustenance to people suffering from depressive illness.

The family

In family approaches to treatment, sometimes called family therapy, the person with depression is treated in relation to their family. This does not mean that the family are held to be responsible for the individual's depression, but it is clear that many of the problems of depression revolve around difficulties in the way family members communicate and relate to each other. Bringing the family together for group discussions is sometimes a powerful way to help everyone to pull together instead of apart, to communicate better, and to help parents develop better relationships with their children and vice versa.

Group therapy

Group therapy is allied to family therapy. Discussing problems in a group helps to combat social isolation, it reinforces for people with depression that they are not alone in the symptoms they are suffering and it provides the opportunity for mutual encouragement and discussion of practical ways of overcoming depression.

Other therapies

Occupational therapy, art therapy, play therapy, dance therapy, movement therapy, drama therapy, music therapy, physiotherapy and gymnastics all help people to develop new social skills, as well as to practice old ones, and to increase self-confidence and self-sufficiency. All aim to provide enjoyment, diversion, stimulation, increased self-esteem and achievement in a social context.

Which treatment is best?

Elements of the three principal modes of professional help available for depressive illness—medical, psychological and social treatment—tend to be combined in the various treatment regimens offered by different professionals.

Although the more severe forms of depressive illness tend to respond best to medical treatment, this is not invariable. About one-third of such patients do not respond to antidepressant drugs and approximately another third are unable to comply fully with drug treatment for various reasons. Specialist forms of psychological and social treatment are not always available, and thus the choice of treatments may be limited.

The best treatment is that which works for a particular individual, and all of the methods described are found to be helpful for some people. If one method does not appear to be working after a fair trial, another should be tried until the patient's depression lifts.

Time

Perhaps, the most neglected treatment is that of time. Spontaneous remission is frequent in milder depressions, and is known to occur in severe depression. The individual can get better anyway, sometimes in spite of the treatment prescribed!

Spontaneous improvement is most likely:

- in a first depression;
- in depressions of recent onset;
- in depressions of sudden onset;
- in depressions following great stress;
- when the depressed individual has relatives and friends to offer social and emotional support.

10 Self-help

IN this chapter, advice and information about self-help strategies for patients with depression are provided. The chapter is written for patients and it is suggested that the GP makes copies of the relevant sections (which are written for the patient) and gives them to the patient who can read or practice them alone or with a relative or friend.

What you can do

THERE are two main ways in which you can help yourself to cope with depression.

1   Try to resolve any life stresses, usually by making some social or behavioural changes in your life.

2   Try various methods of countering the symptoms of depression.

It is important to remember that voluntary agencies, such as The Samaritans, and self-help groups, such as the Fellowship of Depressives Anonymous and other local groups, play a very important role in helping you to help yourself.

Dealing with stress

Depression is more common in people who have had to make major emotional adjustments in their lives during the past 6–12 months, for example, to the death of a family member, the birth of a baby, the loss of a job or moving house. All these events may result in persistent stress.

Over time, the effects of such stress make you vulnerable to depression. In order to resolve fully the depression and to prevent recurrences it is important to resolve stress.

The first priority in tackling stress is to ensure that you are getting sufficient exercise, a nourishing diet and enough sleep. Alcohol, tobacco and non-prescribed drugs should be avoided, they are addictive and increase stress.

Rules for reducing stress

- Get your priorities right—sort out what really matters in your life.
- Think ahead and anticipate how to get round difficulties.
- Share worries with family or friends whenever possible.
- Stay sober.
- Seek information, help and advice early, even if it's an effort.

Rules for reducing stress *continued*

- Try to develop a social network or circle of friends.
- Take up hobbies and interests.
- Exercise regularly.
- Eat good, wholesome food.
- Lead a regular lifestyle.
- Give yourself treats for positive actions, attitudes and thoughts.
- Do not regard difficulties as personal failings or failures—they are challenges to improve your ingenuity and stamina.
- Do not be too hard on yourself—keep things in proportion.
- Get to know yourself better—improve your defences and strengthen you weak points.
- Do not 'bottle things up' or sit brooding—think realistically about problems and decide to take some appropriate action; if necessary, distract yourself in some pleasant way.
- Do not be reluctant to seek medical help if you are worried about your health.
- Remember that there are many people who have faced similar circumstances and have dealt with them successfully, with or without the help of others.
- There are always people who are willing and able to help whatever the problem—do not be unwilling to benefit from their experience.

Adapted from Wilkinson (1987) *Coping with Stress* London: Family Doctor Publications.

Exercise

We all need regular exercise. This might amount to no more than a brisk 20-minute walk in the fresh air. If you take regular exercise, you will be more likely to feel physically and mentally relaxed, to get a refreshing sleep and your appetite will be stimulated. The important thing is that the exercise chosen should be pleasurable. Always remember:

1 to warm up for 2 or 3 minutes before starting, by stretching or running on the spot;

2   to build up slowly and do not over-extend yourself—always exercise within the limlits of comfort (let your breathing guide you);

3   if you are excessively tired, stop and rest;

4   when stopping exercise, cool down gradually and slowly to avoid stiffness;

5   to exercise 3 times a week for about 20 minutes, at a pace that keeps you moderately 'puffed' (not gasping), which is best for stimulating muscles and circulation.

Diet

- Eat a sensible diet to avoid the hazards of being overweight and to reduce or prevent the risks of developing diseases related to poor diet.
- Eat less fat and fatty foods, especially those containing saturated fats and cholesterols.
- Increase dietary fibre by eating more wholegrain cereals, pulses and fresh fruit and vegetables.
- Cut down on sugar and salt.
- Do not change your diet too quickly, substitute a few products at a time and add new foods rather than just cutting out those that you currently eat and that are bad for you.
- Remember, too much tea or coffee can be overstimulating, and excessive alcohol is certainly no friend to good health. Reduce your intake of tea, coffee or cola to no more than 2 – 3 drinks daily.

Sleep

Not everybody needs 8 hours of sleep a night. As we grow older we often need no more than 4 or 5 hours sleep a night. The older we get, the longer it takes to get off to sleep, the more frequently we wake during the night and the less total sleep we have. The amount of sleep we need also depends on the amount of physical activity we undertake and on our state of health.

Sleep problems are particularly troublesome for people with depression, and take the following forms:

- Difficulty getting to sleep even when tired.
- Waking up much earlier than usual and being unable to get back to sleep.
- Restless sleep with repeated waking during the night.
- Excessive sleep during the day.

Causes of disturbed sleep

Stimulants

Much of the difficulty in sleeping is caused by a high intake of caffeine in tea and coffee, as well as in cola drinks, and nicotine in cigarettes.

Rebound effects of sedative drugs

Many sedative drugs that induce sleep tend to act as stimulants when their sedative effects wear off: this effect can be caused by sleeping tablets. Alcohol has a similar effect: this results in getting off to sleep quickly, but waking up within a few hours and having difficulty getting back to sleep.

Changing activities

People who do shift work may find it difficult to adjust to changing sleep and activity patterns. Similar problems may arise on holiday, especially when long-distance travel and changes of climate are involved.

Physical illness

Pain is a common cause of disturbed sleep; in addition, breathing difficulties, a chronic cough or the need to pass urine frequently may interrupt sleep.

Coping with disturbed sleep

It is helpful to make a daily diary of your sleep pattern because this will show you whether the problem is as bad as you thought, and whether it is getting worse, getting better or staying much the same over a period. It will also help you to judge whether anything you have tried to improve your sleep has had any effect.

Record the times you sleep in each 24-hour period. Record the quality of each sleep, e.g. restful, fitful or dozing. Note whether the sleep was in bed, in a chair or in front of the television. Note whether you used anything to help you sleep (e.g. drug, hot drink, relaxation, etc.).

Hints on getting to sleep

- Try not to worry about the amount of sleep you have, this makes things worse.
- Go to bed at a regular time.
- If you find that you have been going to bed too early, go to bed 15 minutes later each evening for a week or so until your sleep improves.
- If you wake tired in the morning, try bringing your bedtime forward by 15 – 30 minutes until you wake refreshed and not too early.
- Avoid sleeping during the day and reduce the number of naps you have so that you are more tired at bedtime.
- Eat your evening meal at a regular time, several hours before you go to bed.
- A quiet stroll in the evening will help you relax and make you feel more tired.
- Avoid stimulating drinks (including tea, coffee and colas) and tobacco close to bedtime.
- A warm, milky drink before bedtime helps you relax and will stop any hunger pangs.
- A warm bath may also help you to relax at bedtime.
- A regular routine at bedtime helps you get into the frame of mind for sleep.
- Try to make the bedroom comfortable and warm.
- Try to avoid reading or listening to the radio in bed unless you have found that these are particularly useful ways of helping you relax.

Hints on getting to sleep *continued*

- Avoid sedative drugs (unless specially prescribed by your doctor) and alcohol because these may wake you up as the sedative effects wear off.
- Try the relaxation technique (described on p. 86) while lying comfortably in bed, and repeat the procedure until you drift off to sleep.
- If you are unable to sleep because you are worried and cannot put your problems out of your mind, get up, write down exactly what the problem is, write a list of solutions to the problem, choose a solution that you can begin the next day, and plan exactly how you would carry out the plan. Do not lie awake for longer than 30 minutes. If you still cannot sleep, get up and find a constructive activity. Read a book or magazine, write a letter, do some housework, play some music or listen to the radio.

Countering the symptoms of depression

Many people discover their own ways of controlling symptoms of depression, without the help of professionals.

- *Is there anything you do when you feel depressed that makes you feel better?*
  Keep doing it (alcohol and other bad habits excepted).
- *Do any of the things that you do make you feel worse?*
  Avoid doing them.
- *Is there anything that you think might help if only you could do it?*
  Try it out if you can.

Miserable feelings and unpleasant thoughts

Negative thoughts and feelings tend to focus your attention on things you do not like about yourself or your life situation. Moreover, they tend to exaggerate problems so that they seem over-whelming and make you feel worse. Although it may be difficult to distract yourself from unpleasant thoughts, it does help to decide not to think about them and to fill your mind with something else.

- Concentrate on events around you—other conversations, the number of blue things you can see—anything that holds your attention especially if it is a specific task you give yourself or something that interests you, e.g. guessing whether the people passing are married or what jobs they do.
- Do any absorbing mental activity, such as mental arithmetic, games and puzzles, crosswords, reading, especially those that you enjoy.
- Do any physical activity that keeps you occupied, e.g. going for a walk, doing housework or taking a trip.

Unpleasant thoughts also make you tend to underestimate your positive characteristics and ability to solve problems. Several strategies may help you to achieve a more balanced view:

- Make a list of your three best attributes—perhaps with the help of a friend or relative.
- Carry the list with you and read it to yourself three times when you find yourself thinking negative thoughts.
- Keep a daily diary of all the small pleasant events that happen and discuss these with a friend each day.
- Recall pleasant occasions in the past and plan pleasant ones for the future—best done in conversation with a friend.
- Avoid discussions about your unpleasant feelings because this is unhelpful—tackling your real problems is helpful.
- Ask friends to interrupt such conversations and redirect your conversation to more positive ideas.
- Always consider alternative explanations for unpleasant events or thoughts—although your initial explanation may be that you are at fault, write down other possible explanations.
- Keep yourself and your mind occupied by planning and doing constructive tasks—avoid sitting or lying about daydreaming or 'doing nothing'.

Anxiety, tension, worry or nervousness

Depression is almost always accompanied by anxiety, tension, worry or nervousness, for example, muscle tension, trembling, cold sweats, 'butterflies' in the stomach, rapid or difficult and shallow breathing, and a rapid or irregular pounding heartbeat. This may be triggered by situations such as a closed space, a crowded supermarket, eating in a restaurant or even meeting a friend. At other times, unpleasant thoughts, for example, of dying, or of possible failure in work or relationships, may trigger such feelings.

In almost all cases, some situations or thoughts can be found to trigger this panicky feeling. Once it occurs, the feeling is so profound that most people want to escape from the situation that provoked it as quickly as possible and, wherever possible, to avoid any recurrence. Many people believe they are about to die of a heart attack, or that they are going mad and are about to lose control of themselves.

Neither will occur. *Anxiety always goes away after a time.* Panicky feelings are bodily sensations but they are not harmful. Wait and let the feelings pass. Practice one of the plans below. Use it whenever you feel panicky.

- It can be helpful to start by taking a deep breath and then slowing down and deepening your breathing pattern.
- Try to distract your panicky thoughts (as described above) because this will stop you adding to the panic.
- As the panicky feelings subside, plan something pleasant to do next.

Plan 1 – Problem-solving

A problem-solving approach, like that described below, may be used to define exactly what the stress is and to devise a plan to cope with it. Although some stresses cannot be fully resolved in this way, there is usually some degree of improvement in coping abilities and efforts, so that the overall impact of stress is reduced.

Put your worrying to a constructive purpose. Rather than endlessly pinpointing your problems, pick out one or two that seem really important and make specific plans to resolve them. You may find it helpful to do this with a friend. Sit down with a sheet of paper and a pencil and go through the following steps, making notes as you go.

- Write down exactly what the problem is.
- List 5 or 6 possible solutions to the problem—write down any ideas that occur to you, not merely 'good' ideas.
- Weigh up the good and bad points of each idea in turn.
- Choose the solution that best fits your needs.

- Plan the steps you would take to achieve the solution.
- Reassess your efforts after carrying out your plan—praise all your efforts.
- If you are unsuccessful, start again with a new plan.

Plan 2 – Re-thinking the experience

- *List every feature of the experience:* 'I'm sweating . . . the hairs on my arm are standing on end . . . my heart is pounding hard . . . 110 per minute . . . I think I'm going to start screaming . . . my legs feel like jelly . . . I'm going to pass out.' Write these sensations down on a card.
- *Talk yourself into staying with the feelings:* tell yourself exactly how you feel, then remind yourself that the feelings will reach a peak and then get better.
- *Re-label your experiences:* imagine you are playing an energetic sport and that this accounts for your pounding heart, rapid breathing and feelings of excitement.
- *Think catastrophic thoughts:* think of the worst possible thing that could happen to you, e.g. collapsing, screaming, throwing your clothes off or being incontinent. Plan exactly what you would do if it did happen.

Next time it will be easier to cope with the feelings, and with practice and monitoring you will find that you are beginning to control and overcome tension, worry and nervousness.

Plan 3 – Relaxation

Relaxation is a useful technique to practice when you feel tense or worried. Read the instructions and familiarize yourself with them before having a go. Be patient and give yourself several tries before expecting the full benefits. It can take time to learn how to relax. Keep a diary of your efforts, so that you can follow your progress. A friend or relative may help you to stick to the task, particularly when progress seems slow and difficult.

1 *Preparation.* Sit in a comfortable chair or lie down somewhere comfortable in a quiet, warm room where you will not be interrupted.

If you are sitting, take off your shoes, uncross your legs, and rest your arms on the arms of the chair.

If you are lying down, lie on your back with your arms at your sides. If necessary use a comfortable pillow for your head.

Close your eyes and be aware of your body. Notice how you are breathing and where the muscular tensions are. Make sure you are comfortable.

2   *Breathing.* Start to breathe slowly and deeply, expanding your abdomen as you breathe in, then raising your rib cage to let more air in, until your lungs are filled right to the top. Hold your breath for a couple of seconds and then breathe out slowly, allowing your rib cage and stomach to relax, and empty your lungs completely. **Do not strain**, with practice it will become much easier. Keep this slow, deep, rhythmic breathing going throughout your relaxation session.

3   *Relaxing.* After 5 – 10 minutes, when you have your breathing pattern established, start the following sequence tensing each part of the body on an in-breath, holding your breath for 10 seconds while you keep your muscles tense, then relax and breath out at the same time.

i   Curl your toes hard and press your feet down.
ii   Press your heels down and bend your feet up.
iii   Tense your calf muscles.
iv   Tense your thigh muscles, straightening your knees and making your legs stiff.
v   Make your buttocks tight.
vi   Tense your stomach as if to receive a punch.
vii   Bend your elbows and tense the muscles of your arms.
viii Hunch your shoulders and press your head back into the cushion or pillow.
ix   Clench your jaws, frown and screw up your eyes really tight.
x   Tense all your muscles together.

Remember to breathe deeply, and be aware when you relax of the feeling of physical wellbeing and heaviness spreading through your body.

After you have done the whole sequence (i – x) and you are still breathing slowly and deeply, imagine something pleasant, e.g. a white rose on a black background, a beautiful country scene or

...e painting. Try to 'see' the rose (or whatever) as clearly ...sible, concentrating your attention on it for 30 seconds. Do ...hold your breathing during this time, continue to breathe as ...ou have been doing. After this, go on to visualize another peaceful object of your choice in a similar fashion.

Lastly, give yourself the instruction that when you open your eyes you will be perfectly relaxed but alert.

Short routine

When you have become familiar with this technique, if you want to relax at any time when you have only a few minutes, do the sequence in a shortened form, leaving out some muscle groups, but always working from your feet upwards. For example, you might do numbers **i, iv, vi, viii** and **x** if you do not have time to do the whole sequence.

Loss of interest, slowed activity and lack of energy

- Set some goals for your daily activities, e.g. meet a friend or read an article in the newspaper.
- In small steps, structure a full programme of constructive activities, e.g. in the morning . . . , at lunch-time . . . , in the afternoon . . . , etc.
- Pinpoint small areas of interest that you can easily perform and build upon them, e.g. from going out of doors into the garden . . . to . . . going on a walk with a friend through the local park.
- Avoid comparing your current levels of performance and interest with those in the past. Concentrate on the present and the future.
- If a task seems too difficult do not despair, break it down into even easier steps and start again more slowly.
- *Reward yourself for your efforts.* Try to have others around you encourage and praise you for every small step you take.

Loss of appetite

- Eat small portions of food that you particularly like.
- Take your time eating.

- Temporarily avoid situations that make you feel under pressure to finish eating.
- Drink plenty of fluids, especially fruit juices and milkshakes.

Weight loss may be an important indicator of the extent of depression, so if you begin to lose weight, seek professional help from your GP.

Loss of sexual drive

Decreased interest in sex is frequently a feature of depressive illness and causes much distress.
- Enjoy those aspects of your sexual relationship that are still a pleasure.
- Explain to your partner that your loss of interest and affection is a temporary symptom of your condition, not a rejection of him or her.

Treating depression does not always restore libido, therefore discussing matters early with the GP, another professional adviser or confidant may improve matters considerably.

Loss of confidence and avoidance of depressing situations

Both loss of confidence and avoidance of depressing situations can be overcome by facing difficulties gradually. The aim is to face up to difficult situations in easy stages, building up confidence to try more difficult situations using graded practice.

1 Ask the following questions.
   Which situations do you avoid?
   What tasks do you put off because of the strain they cause?
   What problems do you avoid thinking about?

2 Make a list of the things you avoid, put off or try not to think about. Arrange these in their order of increasing difficulty for you to face up to.

- Take the first item on the list as your first target to practice thinking about or facing up to.
- Describe the target you are aiming for very clearly in writing.
- Practice thinking about it or facing up to it as often as possible until it is no longer a difficulty.

Practice regularly, frequently and for fairly long periods, depending on the nature of the task. An hour a day, either in one session or in a number of shorter sessions, might be appropriate for most targets. If something appears too difficult, break it down into smaller practice steps or shorter practice periods and gradually build up the practice time. Then, move on to the next item and repeat the process.

Do not be put off if you feel a bit worse to begin with—this is almost inevitable. Be prepared to put some effort into regaining your confidence. It is also common to think that you are not making any progress to begin with, and to under-rate your achievements. Therefore, it is helpful to have a member of the family or a friend to give you an independent opinion about progress and to give you encouragement.

Remember to praise all your successes, give yourself a pat on the back and promise yourself a treat when you have achieved a previously stated target.

Setbacks

Everyone has setbacks from day to day. These are to be expected and you should try to keep your mind on your long-term goals.

- Try to approach the problem in a different way.
- Try to approach the difficulty in smaller steps or stages.
- Try to continue your practice because eventually this will help you to overcome your difficulties.
- Remember that you will probably be more successful if you can make your activities or rewards as enjoyable as possible.
- Keep on doing plenty of the things that you enjoy (but not bad habits!):

  i   make a list of the things you enjoy doing and make sure you make time to do them often;
  ii find a way of rekindling interest in skills that you had in the past;
  iii remember your good points and remind yourself of them regularly.

Making a note of improvement

Do this by keeping a simple daily or weekly diary. The first signs of improvment are usually quite small, sometimes hardly noticeable. A diary will help you see exactly what happened—do not rely on memory as this can be very far off the mark.

Also, we have a tendency to remember setbacks more than successes. Again, it is helpful to involve a member of the family or a friend when assessing your improvement, to give an independent opinion.

Write down what happened

Date	Score	Successes	Technique	Target	Fun/enjoyment

- Score yourself from 1 (bad) to 10 (good) for each day or week.
- Write down all your successes, large or small.
- Write down what self-help technique you were using, what target you were trying to achieve and whether you were practicing it regularly.
- Write down what you did not avoid thinking about or doing.
- Write down what you did for enjoyment or fun.
- Look back at your diary every week to see what progress you have made and to make plans for what you intend to achieve next week.

Index